The Meaning of Illness

Edited by
MARK KIDEL
and
SUSAN ROWE-LEETE

ROUTLEDGE
London and New York

First published in 1988 by
Routledge
11 New Fetter Lane, London EC4P 4EE

Published in the USA by
Routledge
in association with Routledge, Chapman & Hall Inc.
29 West 35th Street, New York, NY 10001

Set in 10½/12 pt Bembo
by Columns of Reading
and printed in Great Britain
by Richard Clay Ltd, Bungay, Suffolk

Library of Congress Cataloging in Publication Data
The Meaning of illness / edited by Mark Kidel with Susan Rowe-Leete.
    p.   cm.
  Based on 2 conferences held at Dartington Hall, Devon, England, in
  1985 and 1986.
  Includes bibliographies and index.
  1. Sick—Psychology—Congresses.   2. Medicine and psychology—
  —Congresses.   3. Therapeutic systems—Congresses.   I. Kidel, Mark.
  II. Rowe-Leete, Susan.
  R726.5.M37 1988
  616—dc19   87–28601

British Library CIP Data also available
ISBN 0-415-00191-9(c)
      0-415-00192-7(p)

Contents

Sickness and health appear to be opposites. They are not, any more than heat or cold are, for instance. Just as the latter are effects of different wavelengths, so illness and health are effects of one and the same life. Illness does not come from the outside; it is not an enemy, but a creation of the organism, the It. The It – or we may call it vital force, the self, the organism – this It, about which we know nothing and of which we shall never recognise more than some of its outward forms, tries to express something by illness; to be ill has to mean something.

(From *The Meaning of Illness* by Georg Groddeck, Hogarth Press, London, 1977, p. 197)

Health like wholeness is completion in individuality, and to this belongs the dark side of life as well: symptoms, suffering, tragedy and death. Wholeness and health therefore do not exclude these 'negative' phenomena; they are requisite for health.

(From *Suicide and the Soul* by James Hillman, Harper & Row, New York, 1964)

1 · Introduction

MARK KIDEL

This book has its origins in two conferences which took place at Dartington Hall in Devon: 'The Meaning of Illness' in 1985, and 'Revisioning Illness' in 1986. The conferences brought together a wide range of 'helping professionals': medical consultants, psychotherapists, homoeopaths, social workers, acupuncturists and GPs. The gatherings were unusual because they did not focus on the eradication of pathology or the pursuit of 'health' and 'wellness'. The emphasis was instead on the possibility of understanding illness differently: not so much as a curse, but in some way also as a potential gift.

Those who came, contributors and participants, had few illusions about the pain, terror and suffering caused by illness – among us were many who had experienced, or currently faced, life-threatening physical disorders – and yet there was a shared sense, articulated in many different ways, that illness needed to be rescued from its *exclusively* negative connotations. These conferences explored the idea that, 'in order to be healthy', to quote from Alfred Ziegler's 1986 seminar, 'you need to be a little bit sick': that wholeness encompasses vulnerability as well as strength; and that healers must allow themselves to be in some sense 'wounded' if they are to help those who come to them.

There is no easy answer to the question of the 'meaning of illness': why a particular person becomes ill in a particular way at a particular time cannot, in the final analysis, be given a satisfactory 'explanation'. Readers should not, therefore, expect to find within these pages an all-purpose 'key' to specific ailments and diseases. This book offers a number of perspectives on illness, which may not always be consistent with each other and which may perhaps raise more questions than they answer. The chapters range from the presentation of theoretical models to naked autobiography, and have been selected for their relevance to all whose lives are touched by these issues, not only to the helping and medical professions.

We live at a time of doubt and global re-evaluation: there is no consensus worldview, either scientific or religious. The 'disease' of today cannot be cured with a universal myth or simple answers. The various contributors to this book offer a number of possible 'stories', each providing a way of understanding illness which counterpoints the familiar 'mechanistic' medical accounts: accounts which so often leave the questions that torment the stricken individual unanswered. Such perspectives do not imply a total rejection of the scientific viewpoint, but they do show a concern with the limitations of objective and strictly materialistic descriptions.

In choosing the title 'The Meaning of Illness', I acknowledge an important debt to Georg Groddeck,[1] the great psychosomatic physician, who wrote an essay with that title in 1925. I am grateful to Patrick Pietroni, one of the leading advocates of holistic medicine in Britain, and chairman of the British Holistic Medical Association, for suggesting that I read Groddeck, as well as encouraging me to use the word 'illness' in the conference title, against almost unanimous advice that any title invoking illness rather than health or fitness would dissuade prospective participants.

The conferences (and this book) would not have happened if I had not myself struggled – albeit in a relatively small way – with illness. Dissatisfied with piecemeal diagnostic explanations offered by the medical profession, my experience of illness began to change. This slow process of 're-framing' was greatly helped by books I read at the time. There is much work being undertaken currently which explores and redefines the relationships between 'psyche' and 'soma'. I am particularly indebted to the work of James Hillman and his use of the notion of the 'imaginal'.[2] I owe much as well to Alfred Ziegler's important work *Archetypal Medicine*,[3] a book which irrevocably disturbs accepted notions of 'health' and 'illness'.

The conferences that led to this book were made possible by the Dartington Hall Trust. I am grateful to the Trustees for backing exploration which would not easily have found support elsewhere.

Notes

1 *The Meaning of Illness – Selected Psychoanalytic Writings*, Georg Groddeck, The Hogarth Press, London, 1977.
2 See, for example: *Healing Fictions*, James Hillman, Station Hill, New York, 1983; *Suicide and the Soul*, James Hillman, Harper & Row, New York, 1964; *Revisioning Psychology*, James Hillman, Harper & Row, New York, 1975.
3 *Archetypal Medicine*, Alfred Ziegler, Spring Publications Inc., Dallas, 1983.

2 · Illness and meaning

MARK KIDEL

Mark Kidel is a writer and film-maker. He was involved with the Dartington Conference, a forum for the exploration of new ideas in the arts of sciences, for ten years. He was director of the Conference from 1984 to 1986, and set up the two gatherings of helping professionals upon which this book is based.

With co-editor Susan Rowe-Leete he is at present working on *Mapping the Body* a book which assembles images of the human body from different cultures and historical periods.

'Illness and Meaning' originally appeared in a very different form in *Resurgence*, Jan-Feb (1985) and later in *Holistic Medicine*, vol. I, (1986, pp. 15-26).

I

Most of us experience the onset of illness as an external blow: 'I caught this flu bug', we say, perceiving the illness in terms of something which has assaulted us, almost at random, from outside. We often, in fact, blame others for infecting us. Disease is a force 'out there' which threatens us, takes us by surprise, and penetrates our defense system. Less extremely, we express some illnesses in terms of allergy: a constitutionally-determined response to an external pathogenic agent. Even where we *do* acknowledge that illness has sprung from within, as often as not we talk of an 'attack', as if our own body were the enemy: heart attack, asthma attack, and so on.

Becoming ill is not entirely unlike being tripped up: we talk of 'falling ill' or 'collapsing', or of 'breakdown'. None of these terms exaggerate the sense of disruption we experience at the onset of illness. We talk of being 'out of sorts': our habitual sense of self is undermined, often from one moment to the next. In many cases we are forced to stop work and to take to our beds: life cannot go on as usual.

Illness, more often than not, prevents us from taking part in normal social activity. We have to give up – sometimes permanently – our habitual public roles. Weakened or immobilised, we can no longer compete in the rat-race. Even if we 'put on a brave face', illness wrinkles the smooth surface of the mask worn in everyday life. It reveals, perhaps shamefully, our vulnerability and dependency. Un-masked, we have to withdraw from the performance of business-as-usual and be nursed like dependent children. It is hardly surprising then, that illness is a private affair.

Our negative experience of illness and its effects is directly related to the highly competitive nature of our culture; a world in which vulnerability, fallibility and weakness are perceived as undermining the roles and goals common to most work-places. Illness, in this context represents a failure, an inability to keep up appearances, and it threatens all concerned.

Seen from another angle, though, illness frees us from a burden which may at times become intolerable. Most of our behaviour 'in the world' engages us, to a greater or lesser extent, as front-runners in the market-place or as stalwart supporters in the home. This drive 'outwards' invites the hero or heroine in us; but every such thrust outwards and every career success bears a cost in terms of forsaken 'inwardness', and it is in terms of such forsaken values that the appearance of illness in a person's life can sometimes offer a timely warning.

II

At the heart of our feelings about illness lie a universal fear of death and the associated anxieties about ageing, decay and change. Illness arrives as a grim reminder that 'all is not well'.

But all cannot always be well. As James Hillman has very forcefully argued, in *Revisioning Psychology*, we live in a culture that over-values the 'highs' at the expense of the 'lows': we run away from depression and illness, drawn to the dizzy heights of 'growth' and 'peak' experiences. The idea of 'human potential' that has spawned a whole movement, is expansionist, upward-moving and goal- or product-orientated. Hillman suggests that coming to terms with one's whole being involves descent as well as ascent; it is about recognising one's own limits, being in touch with one's wounds and accepting one's mortality.

The current popular notions of 'health' are obsessively one-sided because they affirm 'life' in a way that excludes the very constraints that make biological existence possible. The 'wellness' offered by the gurus of the New Age is no more 'holistic' than the orthodox fixation on perfectible health: it is rooted in a view of health that is cleansed of negativity and freed of limitation.

Our desire to be perfectly healthy implies an aspiration to divine status, a release from the bonds of mere humanity. In this, we allow ourselves to be guided by a fantasy of everlasting youth, even immortality, and we run away from an awareness of the natural processes of ageing and death, rather than accepting them as inescapable facts of life. The omni-presence of death in the media – in statistics and in reports of war, accident and catastrophe – is an impersonal fact with no real psychological impact on its receivers: we become numbed. Such 'awareness' rarely fulfils the function performed by the dark and ominous figure which in the medieval and Renaissance imagination walked alongside the young as well as the old. Our fear of death is understandable, as is the essential survival instinct to which it is connected. This fear is, however, often translated into a refusal, a kind of forgetting, which may alleviate surface anxieties and yet may actually disturb us more deeply than would a more open acknowledgment of our mortality.

The threat implicit in illness as *memento mori* naturally sends us running for a cure, the promise of a 'happy end' – that myth from childhood to which we cling still in adult life. Illness (and death), however, are manifestations of the unpredictable, the dark forces which form an integral part of life, and cannot easily be brought under human control. Diseases sometimes vanish as mysteriously as they appear; others linger recalcitrantly, unaffected by our efforts to heal. There is, therefore, something very deeply unsettling about becoming ill, for we are forced into a conscious or semi-conscious awareness of the very uncertainty of our being, a sense that our life is essentially beyond our control. Illness involves an often critical confrontation between our self-determined stance in life and the unpredictable autonomy of Nature.

III

Illness is primarily experienced as breakdown of the body. When we become ill, we feel let down in much the same way that we do when our car sputters to a halt or will not start in the morning. The body is seen as a slightly unreliable but indispensable vehicle, rather than as an integral aspect of our essential being. We cannot entirely escape from our embodiedness but we can dis-identify to a greater or lesser extent, from this aspect of ourselves.

Our perception of the body as 'other' is rooted in a culture which has, for many centuries, drawn a sharp distinction between soul, spirit or mind on the one hand, and substance or matter on the other. The body, according to this particular understanding, belongs to a lower order of things; it is in some essential way inferior to mind or spirit. The 'flesh', particularly in the Christian tradition, represents a source of temptation, and an instrument of the Devil. It is seen as an obstacle to salvation which must be subdued: the body, as the seat of our recalcitrant 'animal' nature, is perceived as wild, unclean, autonomous, unpredictable, even dangerous.

There is still, in our times, an association between 'health' and 'virtue' on the one hand, 'illness' and 'sin' on the other.

Our monotheistic culture has moulded the essential plurality of being into a dichotomy between 'good' and 'evil', 'black' and 'white', and has banished into the body all the 'dark' divinities of the pagan imagination. It is not surprising, therefore, that physical or emotional breakdown – involving a surrender to forces which have such pejorative connotations – should be identified with a kind of failure. 'Falling ill' is perceived as a falling down into the physical, a kind of giving way to the lower (bodily) forces beyond the reach of the superior control of mind or spirit. There are also echoes of this one-sided evaluation of health and illness in the holistic understanding of 'wellness', a state which is achieved through 'right living', a kind of pure or sin-free lifestyle, purged of negative thoughts, junk food and other symptoms of spiritual laxity.

It might at first seem paradoxical that our culture's devaluation of the body should have produced the fanatical cult of bodily health and fitness which has, in one way or another, touched us all. Yet it might, on reflection, be questioned whether the cult of upgrading the body, as reflected in the craze for aerobics, jogging and other forms of body maintenance, brings us any closer to proper valuing of, and integration with, our physical being. While concentrated 'use' of the body may in some cases increase sensitivity to the body's voice, as well as reflecting a renewed respect for the physical aspect of our being, 'keeping fit' seems often to be more concerned with the silencing of uncomfortable messages from the body than with authentic self-exploration. By drawing our attention to the tangible 'knowns' of the body, to the mechanics of muscle and joint, we create a cover-up, a diversion from the deeper turmoil which may have originally manifested as a feeling of being 'unfit'.

The near-fanaticism associated with all forms of body-maintenance can perhaps be understood as a mirror-image of body-denial (from asceticism to Victorian prudery, and from self-flagellation to squeamishness at the sight of blood). This cult represents an obsession with the body as object; a distancing from, rather than an opening to, the essential vulnerability of which the body speaks in its 'symptoms'. It is no wonder that we turn to professionals when the body fails to live up to the promise of perfect health, for we are truly and deeply divorced from our bodies and any genuine re-encounter induces deep unease and fear.

Reichian and other forms of 'body-work' offer a way of 'getting into' one's body, penetrating the 'armour' which we have built up over the years in response to unbearable threat. Breathing, massage, movement and other physical techniques can lead to breakthrough, breakdown and a deepening of experience and awareness. It is never easy though, for the 'descent' that such work calls for is rather different from the joyful 'ascent' which many cults of well-being offer hopeful adepts.

IV

When we get ill, our first concern is, quite naturally, to get well again. Given the feelings that disease evokes in us, it is understandable that we should pass responsibility for dealing with the event to a caste of specialists whose cultivation of detachment is even greater than our own. While we may fleetingly consider possible influences other than the biological explanations given for our illness, we desire above all a speedy recovery, a return to business-as-usual. Orthodox medicine, with its arsenal of fast-working remedies, provides, by these criteria, a near-miraculous service. We can so often just be 'put right' by the physician, who comes to our rescue with his reassuring expertise.

Consumer-style health is about restoring a product – 'good health' – as fast as possible. 'Cure' in this context is professionally defined and administered and is as 'external' to the patient as was the subjective experience of the illness in the first place. Conventional, and in many cases also 'holistic', medicine tends to approach illness through metaphors of battle, where victory is signified by elimination of symptoms, and the means of combat is physical intervention. Though 'lifestyle', 'diet', 'stress' and other factors increasingly come into the picture, they are seen as factors which condition physiological processes, and the main emphasis remains on physical intervention, be it through drugs or surgery.

Although there are clear signs that attitudes are changing, the medical approach to illness is based on a mechanistic understanding of the body, and tends therefore, to treat all symptoms and disorders in terms of physical facts, which are only secondarily connected to the 'patient'. The processes of consultation, diagnosis and treatment further encourage detachment, a detachment which serves the needs of the patient as much as it does those of the doctor: both parties, for different but related reasons, have an interest in keeping the feeling realities of illness at arm's length. The measuring and naming which form an integral part of the diagnostic procedure provide a reassuring ritual for disengagement. We all experience a need for explanation, isolating a cause and attaching ourselves to a recognisable disease-category: all these encourage us and enable us to distance ourselves from the psychological and emotional impact of illness.

The problem with medicine's mechanistic explanations, providing as they do a comforting chain of cause and effect, is that they leave little room for factors that might escape scientific scrutiny: for those important aspects of the illness which cannot be quantified, verified and predicted. Diagnosis and treatment may go some way towards containing the undefinable threat which illness represents, but it hardly begins to answer questions like 'Why me?' which sooner or later, in any serious illness, nag at us all.

Disengagement on the part of patient and doctor is accompanied by disempowerment of the patient. This is a renunciation on the part of the sick person, as much as a usurpation of power by the medical professional. It is, as critics of orthodox medicine have argued, true that doctors hold on to their power jealously and keep much information secret. It is, however, also often true that we co-operate more than willingly in our own disempowerment, anxious to place ourselves in the healing hands of the white-coated saviours. Illness makes us weak, but more often than not we multiply this by projecting the role of healer uniquely upon the professional. We also expect from doctors a caring parental role. Though, as children, illness unequivocally offered us the opportunity to retreat into helplessness – a womb-like experience, away from the stresses of the world – as adults, the possibility of experiencing feelings of helplessness *alone* is, naturally, terrifying.

It would seem that much of the contemporary malaise concerning medical practice relates to a sense of emptiness; an inevitable consequence of treatment which focuses exclusively on the body and symptoms, as though absolutely separable from the person. Yet in turning to 'alternative' or 'complementary' therapies, we are unlikely to escape from the anxieties which make us search for 'cures' that work without us needing to engage with, or take responsibility for, an illness. Furthermore, in doubting or renouncing the reassurances of conventional medicine – which are, after all, based on a tangible efficacy and culturally endorsed – we expose ourselves to a degree of insecurity which makes the 'owning' of an illness particularly difficult.

V

Many illnesses can be understood as the physical counterpart or consequence – the somatisation – of psychological stresses which a person cannot deal with otherwise. Being ill shifts the focus of attention to bodily symptoms and suffering, and it could serve to provide a warning, a call to attention. Yet, it is not surprising that the attempted reversal of such processes – from physical illness back into an open state of psychological, emotional or spiritual 'dis-ease' – should be intensely difficult. It seems to require, in most cases, the facilitation of a friend, counsellor or therapist. And this is not surprising, given that such a move goes directly against a powerful process of repression, and involves a confrontation with the formerly intolerable.

In classical homoeopathy, the avoidance and suppression of symptoms is believed to be harmful in the longer term. Manifestations of 'dis-ease' are merely pushed further inwards by suppressive treatment, to re-emerge later in some other form, usually more serious and recalcitrant. The only real 'cure' and possibility for transcendence, according to the homoeopathic view, comes through encouraging the individual's particular constitutional 'disease' to focus itself into acute expression, enabling the body-mind to connect with the particular archetypal pattern corresponding to the disease and patient, through the use of the appropriate 'similar' remedy.

Illness, in the homoeopathic context, provides an opportunity for personal breakthrough to self-realisation, through the activation of the 'vital force'. Such a process does not evade suffering, but neither does it involve an undisciplined wallowing. It is rather a re-channelling of the creative energies locked into the disease process. Suppression, according to this view, numbs our awareness and freezes us into habitual life-processes, pushing us towards chronic pathological states. We may thus be able to cope with everyday demands, but at the expense of not being able to respond to the challenges of life fully and creatively.

Echoes of this perspective are to be found in Jung's thought: transformation is achieved through acquaintance with the unconscious; a deepening of awareness which can be precipitated by illness. The body, according to Jung, is the repository of the shadow: that which is personally uncomfortable, and hence suppressed. It harbours within itself consciousness, transformed through repression, which can re-surface in different form, expressed in the body's strange and unpredictable language. To Jung, illness represents Nature's defiance of our attempts to dismiss and disown areas of personal difficulty and weakness. Owning our bodies is, therefore, no less than owning our 'shadow': everything we find difficult, disturbing or unacceptable. It is one of the most formidable challenges that life offers us, and it is no wonder that we so easily opt out of taking responsibility for ourselves when confronted by disease, and run for the reassuring detachment of the white-coated professional.

It is open to us, if we choose to respond creatively to the drama of physical illness, to heed the archetypal energies ('gods') in our predicament, and learn from them rather than suppressing their call and courting the heroic 'power' of doctor, healer or NHS. By choosing to 'fight' illness, we defy the gods, who as Jung claimed, have 'become diseases', and this neglect amounts to a denial of the soul and the inner depths which give meaning to our lives.

To 'go down', to face our shadow, is inevitably painful. It is also immensely difficult; for to give shape and substance to one's limitations and vulnerability requires considerable inner strength and perseverance. Such a descent involves the sacrifice of false hopes, a renunciation that demands continuing commitment, and a courage that is everything but heroic. There is often little or no sense of 'getting anywhere', the reward for such deepening process arising instead from a singularly unspectacular experience of authenticity.

I am not suggesting that we should wallow in our symptoms, for such an obsession with the surface events of suffering, and the stance of victim which comes with this, brings us no closer to inner process than stoical denial. The hypochondriac is highly sensitised to bodily events, perhaps half-aware of their potential significance, yet the anxiety which accompanies this holds the sufferer in an uncomfortable limbo between the outer and inner – obsessively responsive to the inner and yet so fearful of being overwhelmed by the terrifying unknown depths, that s/he is held forever at the threshold, unable to give shape and ground to the half-glimpsed world within. These terms, 'stoic' and 'hypochondriac' might well be seen as describing, in rather extreme form, the resistances which characterise our habitual 'normal' posture towards illness.

There is a sense in which illness can be interpreted as a

forceful call from the irrational; a chaotic intervention in a life that is held together by the illusionist tricks of 'rational' expediency and a form of stressful 'coping' that may only serve a limited part of a person's rich and complex being. Our reflex, on becoming ill, will almost certainly drive us towards rationalisation – a desperate but effective measure against the threat of chaos. However, another, perhaps more tentative, aspect of our being beckons downwards and inwards through the descent into illness. It is just because illness calls from our soft underbelly, our most vulnerable point, that we have so much difficulty in accepting it as our own. And, it is precisely *because* of this strong resistance that illness finds it necessary to strike at our most sensitive spot.

Illness makes it possible for us to 'uncover' ourselves; to remove the masks that we wear on the stage of everyday life, but also to look within; to loosen the grip of our own repression. We speak of 'recovery' from illness, meaning that we gain back our former strength and can return to normal life; but we also 're-cover', closing up again our wounds and our bared souls.

VI

The medical model we know best is deeply dualistic, drawing a sharp distinction between 'physical', and 'emotional' events and states. Doctors have, in recent years, become more psychosomatically orientated: many of them now recognise, for instance, the link between emotional stress (despite the fact that this is difficult to quantify or test) and a range of physical illnesses. Many GPs recommend relaxation, yoga or meditation as complements or even alternatives to drugs. This is an important and welcome change, accommodating as it does a new range of 'causal factors', but it does not necessarily alter the underlying mechanistic view of mind, body and emotions. Psychosomatics can remain as mechanistic and one-dimensional as exclusively physically-based systems of explanation. This is blatantly so in models which 'explain' emotional and mental activity by reducing them to changes in chemistry. The legacy of mechanism is less explicit, however, in causal models which recognise the potency of non-physical or energetic realities, yet place these as causal factors within a model which views the relation between 'consciousness' and 'matter' in a linear and hierarchical manner.

Our understanding of psyche and soma is so deeply rooted in a Cartesian dualism which rigorously distinguishes and dissociates 'pure consciousness' (*res cogitans*) from 'pure extension' (*res extensa*), that any alternative view of spirit and matter is very difficult for us to conceive. We are trapped inside a model which absolutely separates 'physical' from 'emotional' or 'mental' events, and we have befuddled ourselves into futile attempts at understanding the causal link between them. It is our attachment to this 'either-or' dichotomy which makes it so difficult for us to grasp the notions of energy and matter central to the new physics. It is impossible to understand the basis of Chinese medicine and its concern for the balance of energy, or homoeopathy, with its reliance on remedies so diluted that the active ingredient is no longer physically present, without abandoning the rigour of these familiar distinctions.

We might explore, instead, a view of nature which does not find it necessary to draw the hard distinctions which inform the contemporary Western view of psyche, soma and illness. It is not, however, so much that the distinctions should not be drawn, as a matter of not losing sight of the underlying inter-relatedness from which such distinctions draw their meaning in the first place.

No illness happens entirely by chance, and while we may be able to identify catalysts such as allergy, infection or environmental factors, our individual bodily susceptibility to any of these may provide clues which should not be ignored if we are concerned with what lies beneath the surface events of our diseases. There is evidence that the body's natural ecology includes most potential agents of infection. When and how we fall prey to their pathogenic power is an elusive process that cannot be explained by reference to external factors or 'causes' alone.

While scientific medicine, which arises out of a detached, objective viewpoint, endorses a dissociation between bodily symptoms and other factors in a person's life, perspectives which involve less of a schism between psyche and soma naturally encompass a psychological dimension and necessitate an experience of illness at a more personal level. If we understand illness as being *more than* a mechanical malfunction for which we may not be responsible, it assumes a different kind of significance: we can experience it as part of our 'story', as an event or process which has, in terms of a life history, a meaningful place.

VII

If we look inward we can discover a complex 'story', a personal drama which provides the ground and context for these events. This leads us, however, to a complex network of potential 'meanings', as opposed to the single rational and causal explanation sought by the diagnostician. Once disease is recognised as having a vital 'inner' component we can no longer explain it away in terms of causes and effects. We find it increasingly difficult to depersonalise symptoms: they can no longer be neatly boxed away into categories or somehow exorcised by the use of medical jargon. We have to start recognising the uncertainty and ambiguity which characterises our inner or underworld: a place, like Alice's Wonderland, which does not obey the rules of logic. Experience in this realm is subjective and the intellect alone, which leans so heavily on objectivity, is not sufficient. There are no clear-cut solutions or interpretations, and distinctions we cherish are washed away in a wave of paradox. Through trying to encapsulate or pin down an illness we lose the ability to get in touch with ourselves, for definition inevitably leads to detachment. We have instead to approach our inner reality through a de-reification process, where our life situations, symptoms and fantasies can be played with as though characters in a story-in-the-making. Paradoxically, such 'fantasy' is anything but the sort that leads to flights: a fragment of our innermost story, given form, can enable us to re-emerge into everyday living more able to be 'with it' and really 'there'.

The language of psyche and soma is not easily translated into rational statements, yet much that is personally meaningful *can* be discovered by opening up in an *imaginative* way to the messages that symptoms embody. Through conscious attempts to articulate this image-play, a 'language' can develop – though only to the extent that we are prepared to let go of our inhibition and preconceptions, and invent. Inspiration may be drawn from the imagery of such traditional disciplines as astrology, the Indian chakras and subtle body, and many other 'ways' rich in symbolism. This is, however, no substitute for a personal 'language' born of frustration and pain, the clumsy articulation from our own genuine and immediate experience.

It might, too, prove fruitful to explore the poetic reverberations of orthodox anatomy and physiology, 'reading' the scientific description of bodily function imaginatively instead of literally. From the site of illness (right or left side, hands, skin, legs or head) to the physiological function of a particular organ (e.g. kidneys and 'elimination'), any number of perspectives can offer clues as to the context of an illness and the possible significance it might carry for us. A person with a 'heart condition' might, perhaps, dwell on the associations suggested by common phrases such as 'heartless' or 'take heart', and a sufferer of rheumatism or arthritis, on the rich etymological background and multiple connotations of 'stiffness' (from 'dead' to 'strong', and the word's relation to the Latin *stipare*, and therefore to the verb 'constipate', taken, perhaps not literally but as an image that might have psychological relevance). The image of inflammation as an 'in-flamation' – 'inward burning' or a 'burning inwards' – might suggest something about the nature and direction of a person's passions or energies. Chronic back trouble may be suggestive of a person's difficulty with the weight of a particular load carried (unwisely perhaps) for others, or the nagging demands of a work or conjugal partner ('get him/her off my back').

The examples given here are only intended to give a rudimentary idea of some possible starting points for reclaiming our illnesses as expressions of our own being. We should avoid making the connections too literal or exclusive, for the meaning is to be found in a sort of 'resonance' with such images. Statements that might capture an insight at a particular moment have no claim to transcendent and absolute objective meaning. While our focused minds will be tempted by the comfort and instant illumination of an 'explanation', it is crucial to remember that illnesses are manifestations of a shadowy multiplicity of meanings, a truth that is poetic, ambiguous, personal and by its very nature 'on the move'.

The 'meaning' of a particular illness is not therefore absolute and does not offer the cast-iron reassurance and certainty that a specific medical diagnosis and scientific explanation might provide. The recognition of oneself in a particular constellation of symptoms may well be fleeting, even if it is apprehended, momentarily, in the form of a revelation. Such experience may be 'fickle' in the sense of an inconstancy by objectivist scientific standards, yet it nevertheless has a potency which asks to be considered with respect.

Illness, which touches us so powerfully – physically, psychologically and emotionally, – may provide ideal ground for the rediscovery of the interplay between reason and imagination, as the breakdown which accompanies disease inevitably throws us off balance, undermining our normal 'rational' existence. We may, thrust on to this uncomfortable borderline, find it possible – if only for a brief moment – to articulate a vision which does not draw a fundamental distinction between the 'physical' and the 'non-physical', but which accepts that the two are different 'ways through' reality.

Such a perspective is not illuminated by accounts of 'cause' and 'effect', and avoids the intractable difficulties which arise from having to explain how psyche and soma, mind and body, interact causally: whether mind and emotions influence the body or vice versa. In a world patterned according to 'correspondences', the particular manifestations of a given illness and specific emotional states are not seen as causally related, but as expressing, in their different ways, the dynamics of a person's life drama, which itself reflects the universal principles of Nature.

VIII

In suggesting that we repress the existential significance – the messages – of illness at our peril, I am conscious of having made a one-sided case. There is a very real danger in opening up to illness. The fears surrounding disease, including the fear of death are, of course, well-founded. While detachment may, from one perspective, seem to cut us off from experiencing our illnesses and perhaps also our being, at any depth, it also serves an essential protective function. The forces present in disease, those of breakdown and disintegration, are very powerful and hold within them the potential for permanent incapacitation, psychosis and death. When we allow ourselves, therefore, to be 'touched' by illness, we do so at a risk, for we open ourselves to the full and unpredictable impact of the unknown.

The shamans and healers of traditional societies acknowledged this, and illness was believed to threaten not only the sufferer but the entire community to which he or she belonged. The sick person's soul might have to be rescued from the 'other' or 'underworld' and this task was regarded as highly dangerous, requiring rigorous training, and initiation. Illness had to be handled at arm's length. In the light of these traditional perspectives, the detachment cultivated by scientific medicine makes good sense, for it clearly responds to a universal human desire to hold Nature's chaotic and unpredictable forces at bay. Scientific medicine recognises the danger of infection, and the need to isolate the 'healthy' from the 'sick'. While it is obvious that such isolation serves to prevent the spread of germs, it serves also, less consciously, to protect us from emotional or psychological 'contamination'.

In many traditional cultures, there is clear evidence of a belief in an intimate relationship between individual illness and the integrity of the community. It is as though, when individuals fall ill, they perform an essential function for those around them, invoking the delicate relationship that exists between the established order and the forces of chaos, reconnecting the two. It is though the illness represented a gaping hole in the fabric of conscious life, a sort of leakage, both from and to, the primeval chaos beyond. Illness, in these terms, is creative – it 'speaks' with a wisdom of otherness, transcending the limited understanding of individual and/or community. It is also profoundly dangerous, not only to the individual, because it opens up a sort of black hole, gesturing towards the unknown and unknowable, threatening to undermine the precarious platform which has been established over the abyss of Nature.

The Navajo healing ceremony involves the making of a complex sand-painting which represents, symbolically, the re-creation of the universe; the recreation of order out of the primeval state of chaos. Perhaps it is not surprising then, that few of us can walk away from an intimate confrontation with death or serious disease, and plunge straight back into the mundane tasks of daily life, unshaken.

In our own culture, unable to control the destructive aspects of Nature, we have tried, at the very least, to distance ourselves from the threat of breakdown and decay which shadows our every move. It would seem, however, that this process of containment and isolation may have swung too far. Our survival instincts lead us to shy away from contact with illness, insanity and death. Yet we would seem equally to require some form of contact with these aspects of life in order to be able to be mindful of what it *is* to be alive.

For us, as individuals, the experience of facing illness squarely and openly may, in a paradoxical way, give us new life. By throwing us off balance, the situation takes us to a kind of edge, a point at which, like the Navajo with their sand-paintings, we have to re-create our lives, even if this means abandoning hopes and accepting constraints.

There is undoubtedly a need to 're-frame' the concepts of 'illness' and 'health'. While it is important that we keep in mind the tragic human impact of disease, illness remains *wholly* meaningless within the context of a worldview which makes mutually exclusive and rigid divisions between the 'light' and the 'dark', the 'healthy' and the 'sick'. This approach excludes the possibility that negative and positive poles may, paradoxically, contain each other; that illness may sometimes nurture within itself the seeds of healing, or that an obsessive striving for 'wellness' may somehow unconsciously invoke its very opposite.

As the polar opposite of an idealised notion of perfectible health, disease can only be perceived as a curse, an enemy of well-being. But the ideal of 'wellness' offers a promise which can never be fulfilled: one of those ever-receding horizons so familiar to our 'progress'-biased civilisation.

We are psychologically addicted to the notion of progress, a brighter future and a 'happy end'. Yet a reconciliation with illness both allows for and depends upon an acceptance of all-embracing cycles rather than an upwardly-mobile curve that leads inexorably from worse to better, from grim past to golden utopia. Within a whole that encompasses all possibilities, positive and negative, there is no question that disease has a place. And as long as we chase exclusively after 'health', we shall, in an important sense, not be truly alive.

3 · Items and motion

PETER TATHAM

Peter Tatham qualified as a medical doctor in 1959. He worked in
various medical specialities before working for nine years as a general
practitioner. Having become more interested in the psychological
components of somatic medicine, he then retrained – between 1975
and 1978 – at the C. G. Jung Institute in Zurich. Since then he has
worked in Cheltenham as an analyst and psychotherapist, mostly in
private practice, but also part-time with the National Health Service.
For 15 years, until 1986, he helped organise and chaired the annual
Arts and Therapy conference sponsored by the Champernowne
Trust. He has lectured widely on the subjects of Jung, psychotherapy,
arts therapies, and the psyche-soma connection. He has four
daughters, from two marriages.

'Items and Motion', which makes a link between the models suggested by C. G. Jung and systems theory, offers a way of 're-framing'
illness which has both theoretical and personal implications.

First things first. *Is* there such a thing as the meaning of illness?
And if there is, will it be a single meaning for each individual
illness, or are there several? What does 'meaning' signify in any
case? Moreover, what is illness, for that matter? Could it also
be meaningless? Which leads me to ask: why bother to search
for a meaning? What good can it do? In this paper, I shall try
to answer those questions – though not necessarily in the order
that I have asked them.

Meaning implies significance and purpose. It stems from the
Indo–European root *men-, to revolve in the mind or think, as
do many other words in common usage, such as memory,

mention, mania, demented and mind. The mind, in much of our everyday speech, is given the status of an organ in which thoughts take place. We now associate mind, in a way that is only partly understood, with the physical brain, though in other eras, conscious activity has been associated with other parts of the body. Yet mind is also clearly differentiated from, even opposed to, the material world; over which it may triumph, or strike a compromise, or alternatively be over-powered. On this understanding, mind is the instrument through which we can discover meaning, and therefore it is to mind that we should look in order to find the significance of illness. It may be, however, that there are other possible understandings of mind and therefore meaning, as will become evident.

If mind is to operate upon the state of 'being ill', and find its meaning, then what is 'illness'? Illness is the opposite of wellness. It is 'un-health', and reckoned to be a bad, noxious, or troublesome condition. We experience this as an impingement of disease upon body, or mind. Yet, since illness is most often defined as an absence of healthiness, the nature of that state must also be considered.

The word 'health' is cognate with wholeness, which means complete, or not being divided into parts; and is similarly related to words such as holism and holy. But health is not the same thing as wholeness, or rather that ultimate wholeness to which humans aspire but which will never be reached. There is, however, a formal wholeness, or completeness, pertaining to every minute of life, and which continuously changes and outgrows its prior state, to provide new 'wholenesses'. These changing states of wholeness are experienced as moments of feeling integrated and at one, rather than in pieces. In these terms a healthy person is not *necessarily* whole in either body, mind or spirit and may be leading a highly one-sided and unintegrated life. Equally, a sick or diseased person can achieve a certain wholeness, by accepting the illness as an integral part of her- or himself.

Clearly, since all of us experience illness at some time, none of us can be truly whole except in relation to it. It cannot just be treated as an opposite or absence of health. There are, in any case, many kinds of health: for example, good health, reasonable health, ill health, or shocking health. Each of these adjectives describes a certain kind of health, which can fluctuate and change, at times, from one of these states to a different one.

Illness could, then, be understood as an individual style of being healthy which helps to make me whole, and which I shall undergo from time to time. By searching for its meaning, I become mindful of it, attach significance to it, question its intentions. This is, I believe, not so much a single-minded search for and discovery of eternal truths, but an act of creative imagination. If I fantasise about my illness, and look at it from various perspectives, making as many images of it as I can, my illness will have more than one meaning. An aching neck, for example, may mean osteo-arthritis of the cervical spines. It may also suggest to me that I suffer from too much pride, am stiff-necked; or perhaps, on the other hand, that a bit more self-esteem would be useful, for impudence is 'brass neck', and can be valuable. In addition my pain might be reminding me of the colleague who is a thorn in my side, a pain in the neck. And it can also draw my attention to a failure to deal with that situation. Maybe I should act more decisively, – with a bit more neck, for instance. Any or all of these might be operating at the same time with the same symptoms. The ambiguity of all this is something I must learn to accept; for all these meanings lead to further knowledge, greater awareness, and perhaps even a change in direction.

In the late twentieth century, we no longer need to be confined to single meanings: indeterminacy applies to the real world as well as to microphysics. Pluralism has once again returned to favour and gone are the certainties and apparently simple orderedness of the past. The new physics, for example, asks of us that we imagine not so much the particles which make up matter, but that we focus on their relationship, with one another, for this is what 'makes' reality. Moreover, according to the so-called 'bootstrap' theory, there are no fundamental laws or properties, but all properties follow on from those of other parts of the intricate web which makes up our universe. The consistency of that web of relationships will specify its own very nature.

In the macrophysical world, the exploitation of one element on this earth by another is increasingly questioned (though it continues): an ecological perspective has developed and has been increasingly accepted. According to this viewpoint, the needs of one creature or group will be weighed against their effects upon others inhabiting the same ecological niche, who may have needs of their own to be fulfilled. In a square metre of a meadow, there are innumerable plants, insects, moulds, bacteria, visiting birds, etc., all living in some kind of balance, rubbing along together, feeding off each other, destroying and in their turn being destroyed or dying. It may seem like tooth and claw competition, but all are, in fact, necessary components in the fluctuating state which that niche represents. Without each one of them, the picture would be a different one. In this macrophysical case, as in microphysics, it is the inter-relatedness between single elements in the story which tell the story or stories.

Ecology is the logos of the home (Gr: *oikos*); and home is where the collection of people known as 'family' live, connected by varying bonds, and with shared as well as conflictual wishes. They exist there in some state of give-and-take. The word that home derived from, *hām*, meant in Old English, a collection of houses, an estate, or village. Thus a *hām* is even more a group of individuals living in loose association, with personal identities, behaviour, and desires. Many people make up the community, with a balance among its constituents, in which each is accommodated with their own personal differences. In a *hām*, there might be as many opinions as individuals, but shared purpose and feuds also.

Neither ecological niche, family nor *hām* exist in a steady state where nothing alters. All are in flux, with each element trading off against the others, as time passes. Alliances and oppositions will be made and broken again. Every present 'state' can be described as an event in its own right: a happening. But when I depict such a situation as being an absolute fact, then I err, for all I have done is freeze the on-going narrative to focus on a single frame. I have picked it out as if nominal reality is more important than the setting, connections and their onward movement through time. Today we know otherwise – or rather, we see it through different spectacles.

It will be plain from all of the above that I am concerned with an outlook that has changed from regarding things and objects to one that sees processes and flow: from items to motion and away from states towards change. Not that objects have vanished from existence, but rather that it is now also possible to see them as mere meta-stabilities in on-going movements. In addition, they are totally inter-related with the neighbouring objects of what was once called 'the environment' but is now all part of a seamless field. Things are certainly things, but they are also parts of systems.

So, where does this leave us with mind and meaning? For a long time the human body – a thing if ever there was one – has also been regarded as a self-organising, self-regulating, self-transcending system, or collection of sub-systems. At no time is it stationary in terms of the chemical reactions which go on inside it to support and sustain, but is always in dynamic process. Even at rest, the body is continuously balancing and correcting itself (homoeostasis). It was C. G. Jung, in the early part of this century, who put forward a similar view of the human psyche; that it was a system in process, which he called 'individuation'. The psyche, he said, made its own consciousness continually from infancy onwards. It consistently regulated and modified its own performance; and was responsible for its own growth. The psyche demonstrates, in current terminology, autopoiesis (self-making) and homoeorhesis (a flow which balances), or in other words, it pulls itself up by its own bootstraps. For Jung the individuation process described the way in which an individual could, by his or her own endeavours become truly their own unique person, and this was a process which would never end, through life. Psychic illness, neurosis, was clearly seen by him as an integral part of that process of self-regulation and change. He described it in terms of a dialectic. Psychic one-sidedness (thesis) was compensated for by an activation of unconscious content (antithesis). The tension between these two opposing states would, if held, lead to a new position of consciousness (synthesis). The same synthesis would in due course harden into one-sidedness and provide a new thesis for which the unconscious psyche must inevitably compensate. It was a bold and imaginative formulation which has proved enormously fruitful in many fields. And there is no reason to suppose that physical illness cannot be regarded in the same way.

Jung used the tools then at his disposal, but today we are better equipped to describe those same processes, using theories about the functioning of systems which have been put forward since the 1940s. What exactly is a system? It is a collection of components which function as a whole in a way that is different to, and more than, the sum of its own individual parts. Central heating in the home is a good example of an open system which takes in energy from the outside and exports it back to the environment in a changed form. Its component parts (boiler, timeswitch, thermostat, pump, etc.) regulate the steady functioning of the system, increasing or decreasing heat output as required or when told to. Its operation could easily be described using General Systems Theory. Living systems, however, possess the additional property of being able to grow, which is, in effect, to change into something or someone else.

Human beings having psychic as well as somatic modes, are doubly systemic, and each of those systems (body and mind) is likely to be the expression of some, as yet indescribable, whole state. This theoretical entity can either be looked on as a condition which unites them both, and of which they are both sub-systems, or on the other hand that each of them is a different expression of the same unfathomable whole. In this proposed entity, matter and mind are as one, reflected in the unity of the environment also. Jung called this wholeness Unitary Reality. The alchemist Gerhard Dorn wrote of the *unus mundus*. In physics, today, David Bohm, describes an Implicate Order. But whatever the name might be, it is a lifelike process which can and will express itself either in mental or physical languages. This super-system will inevitably possess self-transcension as part of its nature. It cannot be described in terms of General Systems Theory, which governs homoeostasis only. For changeable systems, ones that grow out of themselves, it is necessary to turn to the work of Ilya Prigogine and his Theory of Dissipative Structures.

A dissipative structure is a special kind of system which exists far from equilibrium. It does not remain in a balanced state, but 'wobbles', recovering from each fluctuation by an in-built damping down process. Inevitably there will come a time when the fluctuations are too great, and the resulting perturbance of the system threatens its stability. Instead of collapsing under the strain, however, as might be expected, the dissipative structure passes through a chaotic phase, when the connections between component parts break down. They rapidly reform, making many new connections with each other, so that a fresh structure results of a higher degree of complexity, able to withstand the fluctuations which broke up its predecessor. The structure has regained an ordered state, by means of passing through chaos; and it is called dissipative, because it disperses entropy (which is to say, disorderedness) into the environment, of which it is, in any case, part and parcel.

Here we have a model for a system which, of its own nature, grows as well as regulates itself. Indeed, the dissipative structure not only brings about its own growth (autopoiesis), but even makes sure that the fluctuations will occur and increase over time (autocatalysis). The dissipative structure will always move towards the threshold beyond which lies a more complex future, for that is in its nature. The means by which it evolves may seem catastrophic and chaotic, but they bring about a new, 'higher', order.

That new orderedness is, in addition, of an unexpected nature, for it is important to note that at the moment of change, indeterminacy operates. When the threshold is reached and transcension must take place, at *least* two paths could be taken by the system, and no one can predict in advance which one will take over. However, once that moment of chance has passed and a new state is attained, the necessities of self-regulation operate once more. The newly made structure will fluctuate and avoid breakdown – till the next time.

The behaviour of any ecological niche, family or *hām* could be described, using this theory, as can even the flow of traffic on a motorway. The similarity, or analogy, to what I have written above about Jung will be obvious. Thesis and antithesis could be re-framed as fluctuations which in being held (that is to say, not damped down) lead to the threshold of chaos and a new and unforeseen state of being (synthesis). But for Prigogine, becoming is a more fundamental process than being, just as the movie is more important than its stills. Being, in this kind of language, is nothing but a meta-stability on the way to somewhere else.

By and large, humans wobble their way through life, trying to damp down their own fluctuations. Sometimes they are too successful in being, rather than becoming; and then they get stuck in one-sidedness and the process of individuation freezes up. In Jung's terminology, following Hegel, this is the dialectical thesis, but in systemic terms would be described as a fluctuation. 'Illness' may then intervene as a violent oscillation in the unitary reality of the individual, or as Jung would have it, provide the compensatory antithesis. It represents a coming apart of the person's current integrated state, which can only be put right by yielding to the transformation needed. This may be greatly facilitated by trying to 'tune into' the purposive thrust behind those events, namely the 'meaning' inherent in them; and thus moving to a 'higher' state of being. This self-generated meaning, often symbolically connected to the nature of the illness itself, provides the synthesis, which can be described both as a more informed awareness of what has gone wrong, as well as a course of action.

Let us take, for example the person who, in middle life, develops an under-active thyroid gland. This results in a general slowing down of the metabolism, a mind dulled by depression, as well as tiredness and constipation. Doctors would correctly diagnose an auto-immune disease, where the body attacks part of itself, deeming it to be 'foreign'. But the illness may also be saying, in effect, 'You're doing too much and exhausting yourself. You're unhappy about the pressure, but you stubbornly persist with this behaviour. If you won't stop, I'll stop you: bring you to a halt.' Understood this way, the illness has brought a new state of mind into being. But it also provides for a course of action. Hypothyroidism says: 'Why not slow down. Stop thinking so much about those outer things and turn inwards. Hold on to your own things, don't let them slip away.' Of course, the problem is that the ailment is so easily cured by taking thyroid hormone. Very soon, the metabolism picks up speed, and the sufferer can go back to his overactive life, fuelled by Thyroxine. If that is done, then no meaning has been reached in the illness. In Prigogine's terms, the patient has not been allowed to go through the changes called for, in order the achieve a higher or more evolved state of being.

A system which is ill at ease, dis-eased, diseased, is, as I have pointed out, trying to evolve. But our tendency when thinking about the sick human being has been, till now, to see this instead as a thing – an illness – which must be removed or got rid of. Alternatively, by using the image of the dissipative structure, we can choose to see illness as an inevitable part of the process of change. We may then decide not to damp down the wobbles that it entails, but assume and look for meaning, in order to facilitate transcension. The encouragement of multiple meaning will multiply the tension of ambiguity which a single neat diagnosis avoids; and may thus move the sufferer closer to the threshold of unpredictable change. From this it is clear that the dissipative structure provides a better image of illness, because it assumes it as a part of life's nature with the fluctuations which lead to evolution. We do not only have to call illnesses abnormal, bad, noxious, troublesome. They are sometimes what is necessary and inevitable for change to take place.

Such an evolution is one of mind, though not *merely* of mind and it is not *necessarily* one of wellness. It may not lead to physical cure, for the illness has permeated the somatic system, with its own inherent limitations. There may be no turning back. But a sufferer can, nonetheless, be brought to a new and unexpected state of understanding; and this applies as much to fatal diseases whose actual outcome will be death.

If meaning is not sought, or the fluctuations are minimised by medical intervention, then physical cure may very well result, but the individual is none the wiser for it. It is my opinion, for example, that recurrent depression can be seen as an iatrogenic disease – that is to say an illness which follows the medical interventions which are supposed to abolish the condition itself. Those interventions may have done what they were supposed to do, and cured the patient's suffering. But if the depression came about in the first place in order to evoke a meaningful response and bring about change, then chemical or physical treatment will only interfere with the natural processes of the dissipative structure which is the patient's whole personality. Granted that ECT and antidepressive drugs may be necessary to save life, without some attempt also to tease out a meaning for the depression, the patient has found no real release. In due course, a descent into the darkness will once more initiate the search for meaning, which is the only way forward.

C. G. Jung said all of this before, and nothing has changed. Prigogine has, however, provided us with a more modern and elegant, model which is both true to the systems it describes; and which connects human becoming with the same processes in the inorganic world.

Erich Jantsch utilised Prigogine's theory to describe our whole universe as self-organising, and self-evolving. For Jantsch, evolution should be viewed as a 'complex, but holistic dynamic phenomenon of an universal unfolding of order which becomes manifest in many ways, as matter and energy, information and complexity, consciousness and self-reflexion.' And because the way of autopoiesis underpins everything, our world today can be understood as a multi-levelled reality of which every layer is in communication with each other, since the 'higher' has evolved through the 'lower' ones. Now a dissipative structure, if forced to retreat along its path of evolution would do so taking exactly the same route by which it arrived there, but in reverse. So the 'higher' layers of evolution therefore possess a primitive systemic memory, which connects them accurately to their own past. Humankind is truly then a part of its environment (as ecology maintains) because the inorganic world is actually carried around within the history of the human dissipative structure which is me or you. And we are able consciously to link back to that past with our self-reflexive minds by the action that Jantsch called 're-ligio'.

In a process view of reality, the word 'mind' describes the self-organisation dynamics of any autopoietic system. A system which is at equilibrium, says Jantsch, possesses no mind. So if mind is therefore an integral and inevitable part of any system which is in the process of growing, then mind is both transpersonal as well as prior to the origins of life, in evolutionary terms. Indeed, since we are dealing with self-transcending systems, right from the start, mind must be (at least) co-eval with the beginning of evolution.

But, if mind dates from the 'Big Bang' or before, meaning on the other hand does not. It rests with humankind, being the process by which the dynamic of what is taking place (mind) is to be brought into human awareness. Meaning is also involved in re-ligio, whereby the present connects with past mindedness.

Without meaning, nothing exists, because it could never be known; and would have no significance. Meaning is our race's unique possession, by which we have always ordered our present our past and our surroundings. Nowadays, we know that the meanings we attach to things are our inventions, more or less useful for varying lengths of time, till superseded, but not inviolable laws of nature, or given by God.

The same is true of illness, of which it can now truly be said not that it is always 'in the mind', but rather that there is always mind in illness, from the very fact that it is a part of an on-going process. It follows that the meaning of illness is not a single and separate truth to be discovered; but something to be given to, or extrapolated from dis-ease.

It can be noted that 'meaning' is itself a noun, but one derived from the present participle of a verb. And indeed, meaning is not really a thing at all, or not only a thing, but also a continual series of operations by which the subject (me or you) may think about and become aware of the processes she or he is taking part in, at the mercy of, enjoying, overpowered by. If these processes are illnesses, they may very well feel painful or chaotic but they are nevertheless those which lead towards the threshold point for change on the way which is for each of us his or her very own path. It is not a path that is fore-ordained, but one which includes both chance and necessity, health and un-health. Undoubtedly, the meaning of illness is what you make of it. But the essential thing is that you do make something of it. And that will keep the ball rolling – an item in motion.

References

Prigogine, Ilya and Stengers, Isabelle, *Order out of Chaos*, Heinemann, 1984.
Jantsch, Erich, *The Self-Organising Universe*, Pergamon, 1980.

4 · Heart abuse

ELIZABETH WILDE McCORMICK

Elizabeth Wilde McCormick works as a counsellor, therapist and writer in London and in Suffolk. She has an eclectic background of humanistic and transpersonal psychology, clinical and time-limited psychotherapy, and has worked at Guy's Hospital and in the cardiac department of Charing Cross Hospital. She is especially interested in the heart, runs workshops and individual programmes for heart patients, and is the author of *The Heart Attack Recovery Book*.

The images of the 'working heart' and the 'feeling heart' which run through Elizabeth McCormick's chapter provide a bridge between the sciences of medicine and physiology, and the imagination. She is fortunate in having found medical specialists who are willing to accommodate the therapeutic practices she offers in a hospital context. Elizabeth McCormick writes from the experience of this pioneering work.

At the beginning of the US involvement in the Vietnam war, a 'Thirty Minute Theatre' play on British television showed eight people enjoying an expensive elegant dinner somewhere in fashionable London. As the silver cutlery flashed, cut glass tinkled, and smoked salmon was rolled around the tongue, talk was of exotic travel, money made at the races, fashions from Paris, Matisse paintings, and who was who in the City. In a corner of the pink candle-lit dining room was a television, showing newsreel clippings of the war in Vietnam – soldiers being blown up, losing arms, legs, eyes and faces in front of the camera; Vietnamese women and children lying dead after a

34

raid; the camouflaged figures in US uniforms running to throw grenades into rush-covered hiding places full of terrified yellow-eyed human beings; blackened faces under hard saucer-shaped helmets. As each dinner guest paused to dab his mouth with a damask napkin or sat out of the conversation for a moment his eyes turned to the silent screen, to the blood and the silent wailing. The eyes would then return to another helping of caviar or the pouring of the champagne. The chatter became slightly banterish. About halfway through the play, one man stared longer at the television screen and the other guests ignored him, not noticing his absorption. He returned to his food and talk slowly, to go back to his staring within minutes. A thoughtful expression was followed by the loosening of his jaw. The rest of the party went on. The next we see is that this guest has fallen on the floor. No one notices. Later, whilst the steak au poivre is being relished, another guest, a woman, also starts staring at the violent screen. In time, she, too, falls to the floor. No one notices. One by one, whilst still carrying on as if nothing odd or untoward was happening, each guest falls to the floor. Nothing is said. The play ends with the silencing of the guests as the television brings horrendous obscene reality from thousands of miles away.

The play symbolises a split between head and heart, what happens when the two opposite personality functions, thinking and feeling, become polarised. We see this on a collective level in the idealism and rationale of the US Government who sent soldiers to fight on unknown territory thousands of miles away; and we see it in the individual – the dinner guests 'not fully taking in and valuing' what was really happening. When they did finally take into their hearts what was happening, the heart could not stand the onslaught. The feeling function connected to the heart is about valuing. It requires stillness. Thinking is quick, immediate but when we allow stillness, we can take in and receive on a deeper level, in our hearts, the quality and value of what is happening – something which mind and thinking do not understand.

In Western industrialised nations, we can see evidence of this split between head and heart. The Vietnam play could carry the symbol for what is happening in industry, education, government, medicine and technology, and which is greatly threatening the traditions of the family, relationships between men and women and our belief system. We overvalue the rational, logical, binary thought processes which dominate the personalities of our leaders. Psychology, too, runs the risk of becoming too rigid, too reductionist in its search for reason and cure. This polarisation means that the feeling function remains repressed and unconscious, shut away in the dark of the devalued, forcing it to fester and to emerge negatively, in bursts of over-sentimentality, rage and despair, gross feelings of emptiness, lack of discrimination and belief, a void of meaninglessness and, above all, a desperate struggle to stay in control. Marie Louise Von Franz writes: 'The inferior function is the ever-bleeding wound of the conscious personality but through it, the unconscious can always come in and enlarge consciousness and bring forth a new attitude.'[1] With heart attacks epidemic in our Western nations, we are being shown the direction consciousness is trying to go. It needs and wants to get fully into the heart, for us to find a new feeling consciousness. And its way is nothing short of dramatic. When we can no longer take the onslaught of being split and lop-sided, with too much emphasis on ego-consciousness, the body itself has to bear the cost. Alfred Ziegler writes:

> Somatisation is inconceivable unless it is preceded by a 'going astray' of our particular talents. Nature seems to tolerate only a limited measure of one-sidedness, when the limits are exceeded or if too much energy is devoted to one-sidedness, Nature counterbalances the tendency through our bodies, as if seeking a more effective or impressive means of demanding recognition for her chimerical plane.[2]

Heart abuse in the form of heart attacks, heart failure, arrhythmia, high blood pressure, enlarged and overstretched left ventricles, infarctions, embolisms, aneurisms, draw us into a reappraisal of the heart on all levels – physiological, psychological, emotional. We are forced to examine. What is the heart really for? What is it about? What does it mean to us? Why are we abusing it? And why have we forgotten what was taken for granted before the existence of the new branch of medicine called cardiology, that the heart is constantly affected by what we feel and think, the way we live, what we ask of it, that it is subordinate to the brain, that it has a language of its own and that it has for centuries carried the symbol of the centre, the spirit, the place from which love flows like the flow of blood itself, that it is the four-chambered beat and continuum of life itself.

'Worker' heart and 'feeling' heart

In my workshops, I talk about the 'worker heart' and the 'feeling heart'. The worker heart is a pump, the size of a fist, situated to the left of the breast bone, between the lungs. Of the four chambers, the left ventricle is the largest and most hardworking and it is here that people suffer when their heart is overstretched; it is here that the coronary arteries live. Filling and emptying the heart takes less than one second and most average healthy adult hearts beat at the rate of 65–75 beats each minute. We might estimate that the heart beats over 2.5 billion times in an individual lifetime...it never stops or goes in for service. The two main methods of increasing heart rate are through exercise, when blood needs to be sent to the muscles and through the emotions which stimulate the sympathetic nervous system to secrete adrenalin. This happens traditionally in the 'flight or fight' response produced by fear, anticipation, anxiety and also in excitement, joy and ecstasy. The person we are governs the heart. The great Victorian physician John Hilton said:

> the heart that is overtaxed by constant emotional influence and excessive physical effort becomes diseased. This physical and emotional overloading comes from what we do to

ourselves and other people – hardship at work, too much work, too little work, too little love, the loss of love, inability to love, demands which enrage us, defeat us, which we cannot control or which we have neither the will nor energy to cope with or the opportunity to opt out.

Many people think of their hearts as a pump or a car which seems to imply that they view only the 'worker heart'. The 'feeling heart' is the sensitive partner which twins with and affects the worker heart. Images for the feeling heart which have come out of my workshops include a rose, flame, fountain, waterfall, the centre, spirit. The feeling heart I see as being responsible for our being able to feel, to accept feeling, understand it, make sense of it, allow feeling just 'to be'. From our feeling heart, we make connections with other people, from bonding in early infancy to sustained love in adult life. The feeling heart allows us to sense what we need for ourselves, to be open, flexible, give and receive love and affection. It takes us into the realm of spirituality, where love is expressed as belief and religious attitude, where meaning is experienced, where a true sense of 'self' can be first found.

The heart is inextricably bound up with the lungs, the two organs working conjointly. To borrow from the symbolic language of astrology and alchemy, this can be seen as a complete system of air and water elements or the inter-weaving of thought and feeling. An illustration of this comes from Jung's psychological studies of the kundalini yoga which discusses the psychical localisation of the chakra system. He refers to the *annahata* or heart chakra as thinking in the heart. He writes, 'we may know, in the head, something for 40 years but it may never have touched the heart. It is only when we have realised it in the heart that we really take notice of it.'

The *annahata* chakra is a long distance from the solar plexus chakra or manipura chakra which is where there is no air substance and which is the more primitive feeling area. In *manipura*, we experience the heat and fire of passion, likes and dislikes, wishes, illusions, great pressure of emotional energy. In *annahata*, we are lifted up, above the manipura centre, above the intense world of the emotions. Instead of following impulses wildly, we allow ourselves a distance, a thoughtfulness, time enough to begin to experience a new thing. The *purusa* in the heart...the thumbling...smaller than small and greater than great. In the centre of *annahata*, we find the first germ-like apparition of the Self. In *annahata*, individuation begins.[3]

The world we live in today seems to offer little opportunity for stillness, pondering, for that experience of wonder, magic, for experiencing life as an individual journey, not without its difficulties but containing the possibility of meaning, of being in touch with a sense of pattern-making. Man is naturally a myth-making creature. When conscious rationale dismisses myth and magic, they disappear into the underworld, leaving man impoverished, frightened and, when it inevitably rises up from the unconscious, angry at what he has pushed aside; he used all available energy to remain in constant control. Heart patients are notoriously tough. They never give up but tend to drive themselves on to continue furnishing an ideal they have set their hearts upon – whether it is to do with honour, their word or promise, their sense of integrity, perfection, what is 'right' in their code of ethics. They want to finish things properly, to go on to the bitter end. Their efforts are accompanied by stubbornness and pride, they are exacting and demand a lot of others as well as themselves. When things are going well and the person is suited to his task, such personalities are successful in the world and in their own lives. But when they are cornered, by traps of their own making or by life events removing them from a position of control, the habit of toughness and fighting on often forces them into patterns of exhaustion and despair from which they cannot escape. They go round in ever-decreasing circles as they try to 'work' their way out. This rigidity forces other aspects of their personalities into eclipse. In the two years preceding a heart attack, many patients report a gradual decline in pleasurable activities and numerous small accidents. In order to 'stay on top', they give up meeting friends, enjoying a novel, a walk in the country – they give up putting themselves in touch with pleasure, joy, laughter, with all the therapeutic feeling qualities which balance a person's life. They stop having opportunities for stillness, openness. The wife of a heart attack patient who had just died said: 'He behaved as if he could run past death itself.'

When we connect with our feeling heart, we allow ourselves to be, we have time to ponder that individual journey of individuation, we are able to experience meaning, get in touch with our spiritual selves and acknowledge a transpersonal dimension to our life. We are not so alone or afraid. If we have no sense of real self, but feel valued only by a false self, by our achievements, lifestyle, the way we look, qualifications, money in the bank, we tend to make relationships which mirror only this false self, they do not touch us in *annahata*, they do not connect with our real self or our souls. Deep inside we feel this lack, this impoverishment, this unconnectedness and we tend to be split and at the mercy of *manipura*...we rush about lost, hurrying in case we miss something, we gobble the wrong foods, marry the wrong people, don't know how to ask for what we want, we feel the fury and frustration, the rage and impotence of the airless *manipura* and try to live in our heads. We swing wildly from our 'safe' head-orientated achievements to the ravages of fury, envy, self-pity, denial and despair...we ache in the heart.

Coronary care

In our literal age, the heart tends to be in the sole hands of the medical establishment and medicine today is very polarised. We have the extremely fast development of technology in medicine and surgery and the now equally fast-growing alternative therapies. It is not surprising that there is bewilderment among patients. Specialities such as cardiology now dominate medicine and people tend to think they are being poorly served if they are not referred to one of the specialists. Cardiology has tended to concentrate on the development of technology – ever more different kinds of test., inserting catheters and dye, taking pictures via radar, ultrasound; monitoring devices are often plugged in automatically when someone is suffering in his heart. Coronary care and intensive care units are frightening and depersonalising places, full of complicated machinery, long trailing wires and bleeping screens. Undoubtedly in an emergency, they save lives and many people are alive today because of these wonders of technology. But there is another side too. Coronary care units are stressful because of their atmosphere, because of the intensity with which human life is being monitored, because of the specialisation of the nurses and doctors. In the air is something serious, critical, on edge, the balancing of life and death. If a heart stops beating, all personnel know they only have three minutes to get it going again before the onset of brain damage. The urgency is catching, you can almost feel people holding their breath.

Cardiac surgery is now commonplace, a long way from the day on which we all gasped as we read of the first heart transplant performed by Christiaan Barnard. It is said that the coronary artery by-pass graft is now as easy, and becoming as frequently performed, as an appendectomy. And the speed with which people recover after their operations is encouraged and welcomed with pride and broadcast on television news. There is no doubt that the heart is potent, but many people seem caught up in a kind of hysteria about this potency. Medical scientists and doctors feel they must find an answer to the diseases of the heart, they must find a cure and stamp it out as if it were a smallpox epidemic. And 95 per cent of all the effort, research and heart monitoring programmes concentrate on the heart as a separate organ from the influences of the person, remote from the influence of adrenalin, hormone secretions and arousal patterns, as if one thing could be found that would stop the heart from 'messing about' for once and for all. Betablocker drugs do, in fact, have this effect. In 'calming the heart', they make the beats regular and well-paced but this masks the effort in real terms that the heart is having to make. Like tranquillisers, they put a shroud over the symptom so that it is not seen, but pay no attention to what is going on underneath. The heart is not obliging. It is not getting better and heart disease is still the main cause of death in Western industrialised nations and has increased dramatically in the past forty years. People are having heart attacks at younger and younger ages. One man in four can expect to have a heart attack between 45 and 60. And heart attacks are increasing among women.

Nor do the predictions of the scientists bear fruit:

> Predictions based on the presumed risk factors of high blood cholesterol, smoking, overweight, lack of exercise, heredity do not bear fruit. If we take 100 men with the three main risk factors (smoking, hypertension, raised serum cholesterol) only 8 develop clinical manifestations of CHD over the next ten years and 92 do not.[4]

Millions have been spent on programmes aimed at changing diet, giving up smoking, exercising more and taking hypertensive pills to lower blood pressure. Some of the surgery done is very successful but there is evidence that if coronary artery by-pass grafts are performed on people whose artery wall narrowings are due to dynamic causes (exhaustion, hyperventilation, hyperarousal, 'stress') rather than rigid narrowings caused by disease (atherosclerosis), they may be given new arteries and put right back into the situation that caused their problem in the first place. It could be overwork, an unhappy or destructive marriage, the constant threat of redundancy or being passed over for promotion, significant personal loss or bereavement. In Peter Nixon's unit at Charing Cross Hospital, patients are allowed to sleep and rest in a darkened room away from the busy schedules of the ward and the noise and clatter of equipment. If the arteries show changes after being rested, patients can be trained to keep themselves fit and not push themselves beyond the limits of endurance. They are given a 'rite of passage' with time in which to be still and get appropriate help - massage, counselling, training for physical fitness from occupational therapists, dance therapists, remedial gymnasts. This medical and human approach has been known to doctors for centuries, but getting the more 'feeling' and less mechanistic approach generally accepted by the current medical establishment seems to be difficult.

When Meyer Friedman and Ray Rosenmann were looking for funding for their research into the personalities of heart attack patients, they were twice refused grants because they used the term 'emotional stress'.[5] Psychiatrists on the grant board thought cardiologists unable to evaluate anything emotional; that it was work only able to be done by psychiatrists. It was only when someone suggested using the term 'type A behaviour' that the project was favourably received and funded. Their work, now more widely accepted, began because of the observation of their female receptionist who commented on the fact that heart patients must be a nervous lot because she was always having to get the upholsterer to repair the edge of the seat covers on which the patients sat as they waited. After struggling to ascertain risk factors, the two doctors realised that there was indeed a coronary 'type'. The type A person is described as someone who tries to do more and more in less and less time and against greater and greater odds, has 'hurry sickness' and 'free-floating hostility'. Further research shows that this behaviour pattern is built upon extremely poor self-esteem and deep feeling of insecurity, poor early relationships with parents, great loneliness and despair.[6]

Ever since we have known of the existence and function of the heart, we have recognised that it was influenced by what we feel and, in particular, by human companionship and love. Most of us, at one time, have had our hearts beating rapidly when we have been close to those we love or been hurt or offended by them. We may feel our heart will burst with excitement, it leaps into our mouths when we are afraid, turns over in anxiety and trepidation, flutters with pleasure, spills over in ecstasy. It soars when we feel happy, free or can imagine joining in with some great universal event or a beautiful piece of music. Most of us know what it feels like to have our hearts sink as if pressed by some crushing weight after the loss of a loved one or by the realisation of the loss of love. And the heart reaches out in language and imagination ... 'don't wear your heart on your sleeve,' lionheart, faintheart, heartless, heartsick, heartbroken, sweetheart.

James Lynch in *The Broken Heart, the Medical Consequences of Loneliness*[7] writes: 'long before the scientists with the aid of sophisticated monitoring devices, physicians were well aware of the influences of love and human companionship on the heart – perhaps the very antiquity of that knowledge has led us to take it for granted.' We recognise the power of human contact but do not understand it. It has not officially been added to the factors that influence the heart such as genetics, dietary habits, smoking. The word 'love' is not indexed in any mainstream physiology textbook that deals with the heart. Stress, pain, anxiety, fear and rage sometimes appear but never love. James Lynch's work went on to prove scientifically that the presence of a loved one, the calm and caring hand of a nurse, or reassurance by others, could lower blood pressure significantly and speed recovery. Norman Cousins[8] writes of the ability of caring others to facilitate the healing process of the coronary patient through touch, word, encouragement and ordinary language rather than frightening medical jargon. What seems to be reflected in our hearts is a biological basis for our need for living human relationships.

The voice of the heart

So what about love; how do we view it in the 1980s and how does it get expressed? Can the new feeling consciousness that our epidemic of heartache is calling for lead us to a greater understanding and expression of love, the love that is reflected in communication and companionship? Can thinking in the heart be the transcendant function or third position that releases us from the individual and collective polarisation of thinking and feeling as we have known it? Love that flows from the heart is not to do with Eros or with sex or romance nor is it sentimental love written in red satin hearts and spelt 'luv'. It is a love that expresses real connection, that allows a true meeting, that values, that is 'lifted up' within the heart to express the voice of the heart imaginatively. It is a love with inspiration, imagination, image, vision, value, belief; and it comes after a time of stillness, from being open to the possibility of something other coming in; it knows no fear, or ego or hunger or spite but is generous, kind and unconditional. It requires a movement from the 'me' culture that has been the first phase in individual enlightenment in which the image is of men and women with their arms wrapped around their bodies spinning around their own individual experience, to an awakened 'heart' culture where we look up, open our arms and communicate wholeheartedly.

James Hillman writes: 'The heart is the seat of imagination, imagination is the authentic voice of the heart – if we speak from the heart, we speak imaginatively.'[9] Much of our culture has become too literal, interested in fact and cause, in statistics and states of the physical cells; the practice of using our imaginative skills gets left behind in kindergarten and is deemed 'not grown up'. But our imaginative power to create images and develop symbols in our inner nature is what nurtures us inwardly and ultimately will keep us truly alive. This potential is what frees us from the trap of literalisation. When given space and stillness to explore their hearts through the imagination, people come up with many different images. One woman imagined 'a red vase, leaking slowly from an invisible crack'. Exploration of this image, amplification of the different aspects; inside, outside, the glaze, how it had been put on, the nature of the crack, what was leaking, led this patient on an imaginative journey in which she experienced an aspect of herself she had never before realised, living in the invisible crack at the base of the vase. Imaginative journeys are not necessarily to mend or heal, although this does sometimes happen, but to help people become linked to a life-giving soul-making part of themselves that is self-sustaining and nourishing, from which energy and meaning emanate and which leaves the person free to choose what will happen to their hearts and bodies as appropriate.

Another person got in touch with a blazing fire in his heart, at first so hot he wanted to rush and get water to put it out but, later, after standing back, examining, preparing himself and talking with the fire, he could value its force and passion, be thrilled at its intensity and awakened by the heat to discover what it wanted of him. For other people whose images are cars or machines, a detailed description of the machine is revealing and often surprises people who say they have no imagination, that they make no images in their mind's eye. 'A broken down transit van with the name painted out' came from a man who had had eight moves and even more houses in the last two years, who had been made redundant and whose angina had become crippling.

Images can be explored and linked with the physical, emotional and historical life of the person, they can be dovetailed in, and be seen to make sense in terms of the person's life. But their potency is something not fully realised at first – they start people off on another way of thinking and experiencing, they allow him or her access to an inner dimension that can trigger off dreams, other images and an awareness of synchronicity. Putting people in touch with this rich, inner world of imagery helps them to make that movement away from literalisation and rigid focus. It helps them to begin to experience a feeling for self and other and the beginning of love of self.

Love from the heart, a 'lifted up' love, can be more discerning, more discriminate than the immediate, instinctual 'gut' reactions we mistake for love. Because it requires stillness and pondering to be able to communicate with this kind of love, there is time for the world of the instincts to be valued for what they are, not excluded or mistaken for what they are not. 'We all need love so desperately we are vulnerable to its imitations, whether they be found in an advertising campaign for perfume or a self-made Messiah aiming at a multi-million dollar income rather than crucifixion.'[10]

We all need love and yet there is no agreement as to what it is. There are so many different expressions – baby love, family love, sexual love, romantic love, the love of God, love of friends and companions, love of beauty, love of self. People seem wary of expressions of love, and fear a loss of independence if they 'give in' to love. Real love can go unnoticed, and only become fully realised during periods of reflection, like the love we experience from parents early in life that gets masked by the hate and disillusionment necessary for wrenching oneself away from the family to claim one's own life. Only later do we have the realisation that we were loved, in the subjective, limited but *only* way the parent or friend could express it. We can be so clouded with fury at what is not being done for us that we fail to see what is being attempted. In these times we are operating from the 'gut' of *manipura* rather than *annahata*. Real love may only be experienced in moments when we are 'opened up' and 'lifted up' by its potency. The psychologies of blame have tended to make families demonic places for the individual, full of castration anxiety, sibling rivalry and a force against personal growth. Many therapies never mention the word love or admit to its presence, but demote it to a libidinal force that is part of the instinctual nature or impossibly wrapped up in the Oedipus or Electra complexes. This attitude is closed and reductionist, there is no room for imagination, for myth, magic and wonder. It offers little hope.

Love and feeling have long been considered the province of women and associated along with the feminine principles of containment, acceptance, diffuse awareness, intuition and receptiveness. At the same time, women have been at the centre or heart of the family. Women will always be the mothers and it is from good enough mothering that we learn about one kind of love – bonding, sensual touch, affection, adoration, holding, possession. The greatest gift a mother can give a child is unconditional love. 'I totally loved them, totally held them, totally let them go.'[11] Through mothering we learn about boundaries, whether we are good or bad in Mother's eyes, whether it is okay to be ourselves. Whatever is our original seed is planted in the garden of the parents. But to look only at mothering, at the good and bad breast, limits us to that one experience. It might have given us a poor damaged start on one level but, if we allow our imagination to be stimulated, we can find inspiration, meaning and love at different times of our life, in different situations and with different people. We are not limited to the one-off experience of parenting which might have been a bad one – that is not all there is. We cannot spend our lives looking for the mother and father we never had. We need to get in touch with the nature of our original seed with which we came into life.

Since the contraceptive pill and the emergence of the Women's Movement, women have shifted their traditional role. In Britain, 60 per cent of women work outside home and most of them have children. Men are being asked to participate in areas previously under the sole charge of women. But there is something not yet quite right between men and women, a 'new' acceptable kind of relationship has not really been established, and couples appear to be thrashing around in a confusing mixture of old and new approaches. Many very successful women in the outside world have lonely personal lives and secretly long for a knight on a white horse or an engagement ring hidden in a box of chocolates. Some of the 'feminine' type men are unhappy and directionless and find themselves bound up with stronger women who make them feel inadequate and impotent. Children growing up have a vast array of personas on which to model themselves. What seems to be emerging out of this is our individual need to develop those qualities of masculine and feminine each within ourselves separately. What women have often carried for men in terms of emotional need and feeling they must give up, even if it means the loneliness and suffering of Innana[12] and the puzzlement and fury of men. Men, in turn, need to claim not only the feminine side of their natures…that ability to be open, flexible, and compassionate, but also to dig deep and discover their own masculine nature of feeling; something Robert Bly describes as primitive, deeply spiritual, wild.[13] Women and men would then come to thinking in the heart, a way of expressing feeling, from different perspectives…women from the depths of their own being and those of the Goddesses that have gone before; men from the depths of their own particular male journey which has nothing to do with mothers or mothering.

Many of the relationships I see are struggling in a fight for supremacy, control, for establishing who is 'right'. Couples can't let go with each other, they stay on guard, they keep one foot in the door marked 'out', they are not wholehearted. Some men who need to keep their feminine natures suppressed marry women who will live out the needful, vulnerable side of themselves; they end up wondering why they despise the woman they married and feel bitter that their attempts at control, at 'doing and providing everything possible' as husbands does not satisfy them – in fact, can actually make them physically ill, particularly in their hearts.

Couples who refuse intimacy have tried to make a fetish of the 'sex and run'-type experiences, boasting of sexual encounters where not even names are exchanged and nothing is 'given away' or lost. One member of a couple may develop a heart disorder in a desperate attempt on the part of the psyche to express what is happening in the relationship; to make conscious the unfeeling, uncommitted unloving nature of their union. It may be the only way someone can let it be known how much they feel hurt by the other. A rigid uncaring coldness is dramatically unique to certain couples and some are destructively bound up; they cannot give to each other but they cannot give up. Sometimes heart attack brings enough of a shock for people to re-evaluate the seriousness of their situation, to ask for help. Sometimes the attack polarises the couple even more, the patient's partner being suffused with fury and rage, envy and resentment at the care and attention the patient is getting outside of the marriage or relationship, which has not been forthcoming within.

The stoppings and suffocations of the heart force an examination of relationships, both past and present, both inside and out of the personality, both with self and other. Early losses and bereavements which have never been properly mourned, never been allowed to be taken into, and expressed by, the heart and soul, often surface with relief, pain and joy after an attack upon the heart.

After a certain time, I always ask people, quietly, if they knew why they had a heart attack. Everyone I have spoken to has some idea, however vague. 'I knew something was wrong but I just couldn't put my finger on it'; 'I felt that I was stretched out, like being in a mangle'; 'I got so boxed in I wondered how on earth I could go on'; 'I often wondered …is this all there is'. One sensed a deep sadness, loneliness and impoverishment behind these words and an unconnectedness with anything of meaning.

Heart patients who are able to make use of a 'rite of passage' experience to explore what has happened to them, can often unearth different parts of themselves that have been suppressed. They have time and opportunity to express their needs, both practical and emotional, their fears, their hopes, often for the first time in their lives. When encouraged to look at their hearts from both worker and feeling aspects, they can appreciate how each influence the other and learn to be sensitive to the heart's demands. For many heart patients, this is the first time they have stopped long enough to experience what effort really is, how much their demands have overtaxed their heart. I have known many heart patients to begin a completely different kind of life after being awakened by their hearts. It is as if they are freed by their hearts from living lop-sidedly, stuck on a treadmill existence, dying slowly inside. Through counselling, individuals can make this inner journey towards a more loving and wholehearted relationship with themselves.

Thinking in the heart requires that we dig deep into our

emotional natures first, that we face our fear of letting go, of stopping, of emptiness, of being ignored or even annihilated if we behave in any other way than on the rigid path of control. From this firm emotional base, we can then have the assuredness to be lifted up into the heart and into the new heart consciousness and love that flows through it.

Failure to listen to the epidemic murmurings and chokings of the heart forces the collective split referred to at the beginning. At the violent end of this polarisation is the explosive, destructive, fully somatised fact of nuclear weaponry, threating an end to millions of years of plant and animal life. As long as these weapons are externalised, the war weapons of *manipura* – the airless fury, rage and anger at our human frailty and powerlessness – remain unchallenged, liable to make us faint like the dinner guests in the play; not 'lifted up' and connected. If we can stop long enough to really listen to what the individual and collective heart is saying to us, we may be able to change in consciousness to another way of being, and continuing.

References

1 Von Franz, Marie Louise (1971), *Jung's Typology*, Zurich; Spring Publications.
2 Ziegler, Alfred (1983), *Archetypal Medicine*, Zurich, Spring Publications.
3 Jung, C. G. (1975-6), *Commentary on the Kundalini Yoga*, Spring.
4 Editorial (1977), *British Medical Journal* I1302.
5 Rosenmann, R. and Friedman, M. (1974), *Type A Behaviour and Your Heart*, New York, Fawcett City Books.
6 Friedman, Meyer and Ulmer, Diane (1984), *Treatment of Type A Behaviour and Your Heart*, New York, Knopf.
7 Lynch, James (1979), *The Broken Heart, the Medical Consequences of Loneliness*, Sydney, Harper & Row.
8 Cousins, Norman (1983), *The Healing Heart*, New York, W. W. Norton.
9 Hillman, James (1981), *The Thought of the Heart*, Eranos Lectures, Dallas, Spring Publications.

10 Haddon, Celia (1985), *The Powers of Love*, London, Michael Joseph.
11 Client speaking to Author.
12 Perera, Sylvia Brinton (1981), *Descent to the Goddess*, Toronto, Inner City Books.
13 Bly, Robert (1982), 'What do men want?', *New Age*, May.

5 · The doctor versus King Canute: from Georg Groddeck to family therapy

SEBASTIAN KRAEMER

Sebastian Kraemer (BA, MBBS, MRCP, MRCPsych) is a consultant psychiatrist in the Child and Family Department of the Tavistock
Clinic and in the Paediatric Department of the Whittington Hospital.
In the 1960s, after a first degree in philosophy, Dr Kraemer was
trained in medicine and paediatrics at Guy's Hospital where the late
Dr Ronald MacKeith introduced him to the complexities of
psychosomatic disease. He gained general psychiatric experience at
the Maudsley Hospital, after which he went to the Tavistock Clinic,
where he stayed to learn child psychiatry, individual and family
therapy. He has been teaching at the London Institute of Family
Therapy since 1979.

    The cases described in this chapter were referred to Dr Kraemer as
liaison psychiatrist at the Whittington Hospital. The chapter is a
revised version of an article 'Who will have my tummy ache if I give
it up?', originally published in *Family Systems Medicine*, vol. 1, no. 4
(1983), pp. 51-9, Brunner/Mazel, New York. Other publications
include 'A Note on Spinoza's Contribution to Systemic Therapy',
Family Process, vol. 21, (1982), pp. 353-7 and 'Leaving Home, and
the Adolescent Family Therapist', *Journal of Adolescence* vol. 5, (1982)
pp. 51–62.

    In this chapter, Dr Kraemer looks at illness not so much in terms of
its meaning for an individual afflicted child, but in terms of its
function for the child's family, in particular the way in which a child
may – unconsciously – take on his or her parents' difficulties.

Introduction: meaning of illness and function of illness

In 1928 Georg Groddeck reported[5] his treatment of a woman with general oedema, due to heart failure. The swollen tissues subsided after her confession to him that she should never have married, because she had once pledged to become a nun, and had therefore broken her vow of celibacy. The patient passed huge quantities of urine and lost 25 kilogrammes the following week. This wonderful story is a model of treatment through the revelation of symbolic meaning (in this case 'conflict in the heart') and is an inspiration to doctors and other healers who seek the meaning of illness. For many patients, however, such a route is not available. Nemiah et al.[12] have described a kind of emotional indifference ('alexithymia') in psychosomatic patients. These people, they observed, cannot talk about meaning, they can only talk about symptoms. There is a group of child patients who are like this – they do not seem to be very ill but are extremely disabled by their symptoms, which also disturb their parents greatly. Furthermore, there do not seem to be any obvious emotional or psychological problems to account for their complaints. Typically these patients are very nice, even sweet children between the ages of 6 and 13, who suffer baffling, sometimes very distressing symptoms because of which they get admitted into hospital. In such children the capacity to reflect on their condition is very limited. As with psychosomatic subjects in general the symptom is a concrete experience which, though it may have developed from a thought or fear, has become buried deep in the body, not easily reached by a therapist working with the child alone.[4]

Instead of asking the child to think or feel, family therapists working with such patients have tried to see the illness not so much in terms of its meaning for the child as its function for the family, in particular the way in which the child's symptom effectively protects the parents, at least for a while, from attending to their own troubles. The unacknowledged conviction of the child is 'I will make you better by my suffering.'

The urge to heal one's parents, though compellingly identified by a psychoanalyst,* has in my view been most successfully exploited in family therapy because there, together with their children in the room, the parents actually have the chance to challenge their offspring's loyal sacrifice on their behalf – to say, in effect, 'you are right that we are in difficulties, but now we have grasped that, we can manage in our own way, even if it means getting help from someone else. The most helpful thing you can do now is to get well.' While not having a lasting solution for it, the child perceives the parents' problem with painful accuracy and will not begin to give up his or her vigil without convincing evidence, however slight, that they have discovered new reserves of competence to deal with it.

The essential discipline of this approach is the 'positive connotation' of the symptom[7,13] through which the therapist tries to understand how it is maintained by its relatively benign effects, whatever the nature of the cause. Groddeck anticipated this reversal when he said in a letter to Freud: 'The It makes

---

*Harold Searles: '...Innate among the human being's emotional potentialities, present in the earliest months of postnatal life, is an essentially psychotherapeutic striving. The family environmental warping of that striving is a major etiological source of all psychopathology.'[16] There is a historical and geographical split between the originally European analytic/symbolic tradition of Freud, Jung and Groddeck, to which Harold Searles (an American) belongs, and systems therapy, which began in America and has largely failed to acknowledge psychoanalytical roots, in spite of obvious areas of overlap between the two. In the first place many family therapists have had their own personal therapy from analysts and secondly, whether you look for the meaning of a symptom or attribute a function to it, the intervention will be therapeutic for the same reason in either case, namely that *previously unconnected bits of experience are put together in the individuals getting the therapy*, whether on their own or several at a time. This is so in spite of manifestly different goals and methods in the two ways of working. The split may be maintained by the relatively conservative state of psychoanalysis in USA, where only physicians may practice it.

people ill, because it is pursuing some purpose which it finds useful' but it was not until the pioneering work of Palazzoli et al.[13] and later Madanes[10] that one particular function – the salvation of the family, usually through the protection of a vulnerable parent – was given a central place in family systems therapy. In order to shift the symptom, they said, it is first necessary to attend to its virtues.

This is not how doctors are trained to think, nor do patients expect such treatment. Traditionally, for both doctor and patient the symptom is essentially a nuisance to be got rid of. In contrast, the idea of welcoming it as an independent, even ambitious being is not merely surprising, it also exposes the secret magical fantasies of children who believe they can cure their parents.

A doctor who thinks he can talk a child out of this grandiose assumption by superior authority is doomed. As Groddeck said: 'the biggest enemy of medical talent is megalomania'. In what follows I describe my own work as a child and family psychiatrist in the Paediatric Department of a general hospital, and conclude with a note on some landmarks in the literature. First, a boy who could accept a simple symbolic interpretation.

Kim

A 10-year-old Chinese boy was admitted for investigation of asthma, his previous history was unremarkable. He had been in hospital briefly aged 5, with a high fever and he had a cousin with asthma. I was asked to see him because the paediatricians could find nothing wrong with him. Although I make a habit of not seeing children on their own until I have met one or both parents, I had a spare moment and went with a paediatrician to see the boy on the ward. The medical findings were that the examination of the chest, both clinically and radiologically were normal and so was the peak flow rate. Kim was grunting in an odd way, but was obviously alert and attentive when I met him. I asked him why he was here and he said 'because of my asthma'. I asked him to tell me about himself, his age, his school, his family and so on, and within a minute he had told me that his grandfather had died of asthma. This was his father's father and his vivid description of it suggested that the event had been a very important one to him. I asked who had been most upset by the death and he replied 'my father of course'. I then enquired what was this grandfather's name, but he did not know. So I told him to ask his father what name it was, because that was the name of his illness and not asthma. He looked astonished as if I were a bit crazy. That afternoon I met the parents for a moment to arrange a family meeting for the following week and repeated what I had said to the boy without asking any more questions.

The next week the whole family came as arranged, the patient being the eldest of three boys. His grunting had stopped. I asked how this had happened and father said they had just ignored it, so I was all ready to end the meeting there and then when I noticed that the youngest child was playing with a toy coffin with a plastic skeleton inside it. So we had a short discussion about the children's different ways of sharing their father's grief, but as Kim began to grunt again I thought I should leave well alone. I hoped that now the connection was made the parents would not need to react as if their child was suffering from some mysterious illness. It is not in fact possible to ignore a symptom in yourself or in your children unless you can account for it in some way, otherwise the parents in this case would have done so before the boy's admission.

Unless it was a coincidence that the symptoms stopped after my brief meeting with the child, I suggest that what made it possible for the parents to ignore the symptoms was that a connection had been made between it and something that mattered to them all very much and which they could now attend to, so that the symptoms became superfluous. In this case the connection was made by giving a new name to the boy's grunting so that it was no longer a mysterious problem that they could do nothing about, but was instead to be seen as something normal, however painful, which they would now be able to deal with. After all, grandfather had been dead for over a year.

The symptom as smokescreen

When making a diagnosis of psychosomatic disorder, John Apley and Ronald MacKeith[1] always emphasised the importance of establishing positive evidence of psychological or emotional stress. It was not sufficient, they said, simply to find no evidence of organic disorder in the child. In my view this is easier said than done. Most doctors are familiar with the tense silence you can get when, having failed to find any physical disease, you start to search for emotional problems in these patients or in their families. These children have no idea what is worrying them and quite often, neither have their parents. Nor should this be very surprising. There is quite a lot of support for the view that a symptom which has an emotional origin can operate effectively as a screen for the emotions that started it, so that they are really blotted out by the symptom. For example, if you are worried about something and you get a terrible headache because of it, you forget about whatever it was and worry about the headache instead. Although he was not previously aware of it, Kim was unusually helpful and forthcoming in that he made the connection himself between his symptom and a critical development in the family's life cycle, in this case a bereavement; but notice that I did not ask him about any problem he might have.

A useful piece of research by R. H. Crossley[3] shows, amongst other things, that children admitted to hospital with abdominal pain, but who turn out not to have appendicitis (or any other organic disease) have many more family problems than those with appendicitis. The sort of problems he means are: serious quarrelling between the parents, severe mental or physical illness in one of the parents, chronic handicap in one of the siblings, and father living or working away from home most of the time. So in some cases, the presence of other problems is relatively easy to detect, although you may have a hard time making the link between them and the symptoms you are being asked to treat. But in the kind of case I am describing you do not find problems like these. The family atmosphere seems to be very nice and nobody wants to complain about anything, except of course about the symptom.

If you do ask what possible stresses or anxieties might be affecting the child, sometimes the parents would have a theory about difficulties at school, that the child had been bullied for example. They may have even considered changing school, but very rarely, in my experience, will they volunteer difficulties in the family itself. Yet the difficulties are there and are not hard to find. One reason why they are not considered relevant is that they are just normal processes, like the death of a grandfather for example. I am talking about stages in the family's life cycle. Beginning with the engagement of a couple, the cycle passes through quite obvious steps: the births of successive children, their passage through school, the ageing and death of grandparents, the children's departure from home one by one – often through marriage, the promotion of the parents to grandparents as the next generation appears, and so on. Many of these events are naturally celebrated quite openly but some, like the mid-life experiences of parents as they begin to assess their own lives and relationships, are less easy to mark, and others, like retirement from work, are obviously tinged with sadness.

It is precisely because these are natural events that they do not come into people's minds when they are asked if there is anything that could be worrying the child but, as I am trying to show, it is a good strategy to try to make a link between the child's symptoms and these essentially normal difficulties of family reorganisation. Of course, it is possible to search for and to find more sinister processes, such as deep dissatisfaction in the parents' marriage, or even a depressive state in one of the parents. It is not very easy, however, to know what to do about these things. Parents, quite reasonably, are inclined in any case to put up a resistance to looking at their own problems, since it is their child they have brought for treatment, and they do not expect to be offered treatment themselves. What I am trying to say is that the psychiatrist is likely to be more successful if the child's stubborn and insoluble problem is linked not to an equally insoluble parental problem, but to something which, though it may be a serious difficulty for them, offers the parents a chance to demonstrate their superior competence in dealing with it, once the connection is made. My submission is that Kim's grunting stopped when he realised that one of his parents could survive the loss of a father. Because he could not imagine how he himself could survive such a loss, he assumed with the egocentricity of a child that no one else could either. His symptom in an absurd and self-defeating way served to keep the grandfather alive, though of course the boy was not thinking of this at all. Actually, the parents did not have to do anything to prove that they could cope, except that they were able to ignore his grunts which they had not been able to do before.

Although these connections between symptom and family life event may seem obvious to an outsider like myself, there are several good reasons why they are not obvious to the family. Firstly, the symptom, if it has held the family in its sway for weeks or even months, has done its job well and put other anxieties in the shade. Secondly, these anxieties are often not discussed in front of the children in any case, so the parents quite reasonably assume that the sick child knows nothing of them. The third and, in some ways, the most powerful reason why the family are unable to think of any problem that might have triggered the psychosomatic symptom, is that the *problem has often not yet occurred but is still in the future*, so although they can tell you about the engagements of the elder children or the illness or deaths of the grandparents, it may not yet have dawned on them what fundamental changes these will eventually bring to the family. But anxiety about these changes is revealed to the children in all sorts of subliminal ways.

The psychosomatic symptom in such cases is all alone ahead of the field. Even its owner, the child, cannot say what is going on, but the symptom has become a sort of early warning device for the family as a whole. In the short term this works quite well so that any anxieties about the future are quickly replaced by anxieties about the child. The symptom literally takes everyone's mind off other problems. But time and development wait for no one, and any attempt to turn the clock back, or to hold it still, will eventually collapse.

Casting the symptom in this light reaches in a very compelling way the grandiose notions of these loyal and conscientious children, who at some level secretly believe that it is possible to control time and resist changes that are in fact inevitable. In addition, and more important for the effectiveness of this therapeutic strategy, it also gives the parents a chance to show that they know better than the children about the passage of time and that they can learn to deal with their own difficulties.

So it is definitely not a good idea to suggest to the parents in these cases that their child has a tummy pain because he misses his grandfather or because he doesn't want his big sister to leave home and get married. When parents have become demoralised and defeated by a child's persistent complaints, it is not helpful to suggest that the child will recover if a dead relative is brought back to life, or someone's marriage plans are halted. Some families are so desperate that they might even try to do something like that to placate the child, as if such things were really possible. These attempts only increase the child's anxiety and reinforce his omnipotent belief that he can stop the world.

I want to emphasise that this way of looking at psychosomatic problems is hardly likely to be the whole story. For me, however, it is the most effective one to use in clinical practice. I think it important to say this because I am often asked by paediatric colleagues: 'how do you know that this is what has caused the problem?' My answer is that I am not looking for causes but for solutions and that I am not so much concerned about how the child got into this state, but about how the parents can get him out of it. There is always an aspect of a child's symptom that depends on how well he thinks his parents can cope with him, so that when he sees that they know what to do with him when he is ill, he is less anxious than when he sees that they do not.

Avoiding a power struggle with patient and parents

There are several strategic advantages in this approach, the first of which is that it brings into focus aspects of the problem that no one is likely, up to that moment, to have thought of. The idea that symptoms are helpful (though obvious in the sense that a productive cough is helpful to the lungs) seems to come as a surprise to most people, who think that the doctor's job is simply to remove it, rather than find a good reason for having it. So there is an element of novelty, even shock, which is important in cases where rigid patterns of behaviour have been established, with a lot of bad feeling building up around them in the family. The other advantage of this method is that it protects you, the doctor, from joining in this negative game and behaving as if you were the victim of some kind of deception, as if the patient was playing a mischievous trick on you.* However well you try to conceal it, there is always a risk of reacting with irritation, even with contempt, when faced with problems like these. It is hard to resist the feeling that the child is just putting it on. Any strategy that keeps you from challenging the child directly or, even worse, telling him off, is likely to be helpful. I suppose there are cases of malingering in children, but they are very rare and rather sinister. Just as it is futile to blame the child for his symptom, so it is ruinous to blame the parents, and the third advantage of this approach is that it forces you to go for the strengths of the parents, rather than their weaknesses.

I am sure that most clinicians have felt intense irritation with the anxious or over-protecting parents of these children and

---

*The fact is, the patient is playing some kind of trick on himself and is miserably stuck with it, for at some level he does not dare to get well. I think this powerful sense of duty or compulsion to be ill is probably more widespread in psychopathology than many doctors realise. Failure to recognise the patient's obligation to be ill, as Groddeck repeatedly observed, must account for many therapeutic failures in medicine and psychiatry.

wanted to say something like 'if only you would just leave the child alone' or 'if only you would be firmer with him' or 'if only you would stop bringing him into your marital relationship' and so on.

As far as I know, talking like that is ineffective mainly because the family already know, even if they cannot put it into words, that they are trapped in these frustrating and repetitive ways and are quite unable to free themselves.

If the finger of blame is to be pointed at anyone, it is not at the parents, nor at the child, but at the symptom itself, because what is being attributed to it is an ambition of impossible proportions, like King Canute's attempts to turn back the tide.[*] But before challenging the authority of the unfortunate symptom, it is necessary to bring it to life and to define it as an independent force, with wishes and intentions of its own. One way of doing this is to welcome it as if it were, or belonged to, a separate and perhaps powerful member of the family, previously unrecognised as such. Taking this line allows me to pay respect to the symptom and to say to the child: 'I know that your pain has a very important reason for being there, and we shall have to give it a name, and see if we can try and find out what it has to say in reply. At the moment it is only saying one thing, and you and the rest of the family must be really fed up with that by now.'

This is an attempt to dislodge the symptom from within the child and to introduce the idea that it is the symptom itself that is the one who needs help, because it has not been successful enough in its very important task. The trouble is that the symptom has not been very imaginative up to now, all it has been able to do is to groan monotonously. So I offer to coach it, to enlarge its repertoire, and help it to succeed.

For me this is an opportunity to do some clowning with the child, perhaps to call out to the pain in the belly and wait for a

---

[*]According to Michael Pickering,[15] King Canute never tried to do this. 'His intention was to demonstrate to a sycophantic court that he could *not* control the tides.'

reply, pretending to just hear something very faint but not clear enough to understand, or to be mockingly respectful and subservient to it like a court jester with his king. In any case with children of this age and personality it is not usually difficult to engage them in play like this with some immediate if temporary relief for them, because they usually have to be very serious about their pain and do not let themselves or their symptoms go very easily.

It is important to emphasise that this playfulness is not intended to distract the child from his preoccupations and the pain; that would simply not work, or not for long anyway. The idea, on the contrary, is to go along wholeheartedly with the child's earnest and necessary attachment to his symptom and to play with that fact, knowing that at some level he is doing the right thing by harbouring it. As far as I know it was Groddeck who first said that the patient is always right. So this playing with the child is not anything that could be called reassurance in the usual sense. I am sure that reassurance *is* a powerful piece of medical equipment, but in these cases it is clearly insufficient, otherwise I can assume that the paediatricians would have done so already and no psychiatric referral would have been necessary.

Safia

Here is a case that illustrates some of these points. The patient is a Pakistani girl of 9 who was referred to me after an urgent admission to the ward for investigation of abdominal pain. She had a history of ureteric reflux, which had been diagnosed when she was 2, and for which she had been on prophylactic antibiotics since then. There had been two hospital admissions for urinary tract infections, one when she was 5 and the other when she was 7 years old. Three months prior to this referral she had had that mysterious condition Bell's Palsy, which had fortunately completely remitted with steroid treatment. All medical investigations on this occasion were negative and I saw the child in a side room off the ward, together with her parents and the paediatrician. What emerged was what I now regard as a classical picture, the patient being one of the younger children in a family where the eldest are leaving home and getting married, and where there is illness in one or more grandparents.*

In this particular family the patient is the youngest of four girls: the eldest has left home and is recently married; the second eldest has married and has a child, still lives at home but is planning to emigrate. The father is a successful businessman, a member of an aristocratic caste in the Pakistani hierarchy, and the mother is a housewife who does not work outside the home. After an enquiry about the pain and the family's reactions to it, I asked about the rest of the family and heard about the two eldest sisters. I asked Safia which parent would miss the eldest children the most and she said, without any hesitation, that mother would since, as father was so often away on business, she relied on them so much for company. I also heard that the father's mother was quite ill in Pakistan and that both parents were naturally worrying about that. I suggested that the pain this child had was like a very busy person that wanted to do all sorts of jobs, like being a doctor for the grandmother, and a companion for the mother.

*My clinical impression is that these families with physical symptoms have had more than their fair share of premature deaths, particularly in the grandparental generation. (In the Pakistani family, father lost *his* father when he was 14. Mother lost hers when she was 20. All three older brothers of father are dead, the third having been murdered.) The connection could be that parents who miss a developmental stage through illness or death of their parents have difficulty in handling that stage in their children. As a preliminary study it should not be difficult to compare the rates of early grandparental death in populations of child psychiatric, paediatric, and control children. There are studies showing the connection between childhood illness and recent life events[2] and an important one relating *onset* of diabetes mellitus to parental loss by death or marital disruption.[9] Froma Walsh has linked schizophrenia with grandparent death.[17] Thus it is a good idea to make a three-generation family tree a routine part of history-taking.

Accordingly, I told Safia to give her pain a chance as it was clearly confused and over-worked. Each day of the week, at a set time which she arranged with her parents, she would sit with her mother for half an hour and practise having the pain, which was to be devoted to a separate duty each night of the week.

With this task I was trying to get the family to behave differently towards the pains by instructing them to do something together which actually dramatises the symptom's protective function for them, particularly for the mother.

The child took a pencil and paper and wrote down all these tasks very diligently and we had a lot of fun arranging it. This meeting, which lasted over an hour, concluded with Safia being discharged from hospital and another appointment was made to see me two weeks later. However, ten days after our meeting she was re-admitted and I arranged to see the family on the ward as soon as I could. This time I took more trouble to find out what actually happened when she got the pain. The pattern was stunningly familiar; she would be taken into bed with her parents. We talked about the pain again and I asked her what it should be called and what animal it would be like. She gave it the name Timmy and said he was a bear. The fact that it was a male immediately led father to talk of his desire for a son; they had had two daughters, then after a gap of nine years had planned to have another child. They had a third girl and finally yet another, our patient with the pain. For this proud, aristocratic Islamic man no son was quite a blow, so I could say that the pain was a royal pain (the joke was lost on the family) that was trying to be a boy for the father, which he clearly now would never have. But the next stage was the most important: I advised Safia that Timmy was too much for her to deal with and that she should give him to the parent of her choice, whichever she thought would be best able to cope with him. So when she had a pain during the night she was to go to her parents' room, leave it there and return to bed.

Father got into the spirit of this right away and announced

with finality that his daughter had stolen his pain and that he wanted it back, she had no right to keep it, he and his wife could take care of it themselves. I thanked the father for his innovative idea and soon we ended the session. Again I should say that these sessions lasted well over an hour, so that I am summarising quite drastically.

At the follow-up meeting a month later only father and daughter attended and they reported, in father's words, '95 per cent improvement' in the pains. A further follow-up meeting two months later showed that there had been only one bad episode of pain and the child had been seen in casualty, only to be sent home immediately because she was already well.

I think my earlier intervention was a failure, firstly because I did not attend well enough to the family's actual and regular way of responding to the symptom and, secondly, because father had been given nothing to do, yet was clearly deeply involved and very keen to take an active part. If parents find that there is something that they can do to effect a change in the symptom then there is a chance that one of the child's principal anxieties, namely that the parents are not going to be able to cope, is eased and the symptom diminishes; this sets up a benign spiral in place of the vicious one that preceded it.

In the two examples I have mentioned, there were symptoms which had no diagnosis except that they were suitable for referral to a child psychiatrist. This is not a very respectable problem to have. To say that a symptom, especially a pain, is psychosomatic or psychological is a very damning diagnosis because it is so often misunderstood to mean that the patient is putting it on for some mischievous purpose. So there is an urgent need to reverse that impression and allow the child gracefully to give it up. The method I have outlined here involves making a link between the problem and an important development in family life, so that a positive function is found for the symptom that at one and the same time gives it a respectable pretext for having been there, and a good enough reason to disappear, since there are obviously better ways of being helpful to your parents than suffering from a mysterious illness.*

Although I cannot always expect parents to be as inspired as Safia's father, interventions like these are successful if the family discovers through them new ways of dealing with the dilemmas that they face. I do not think this discovery is always a conscious one, which is why it seems better to recommend various tasks for the family, which they may not see the significance of, but are still willing to try out. Because I have this theoretical viewpoint, it is tempting to offer the family explanations along these lines, and sometimes they make sense, but explanations do not readily lead to enlightenment in this type of problem, and I think we have to accept that there are other ways of discovering solutions to psychological problems than through thought. Without having told them in so many words, I believe the final intervention with the Pakistani family was effective because it hinted to the parents that they could be a couple still, even though the coupling of the mother with the older daughters was coming to an end, or at least changing in a very dramatic way. The youngest girl could learn that she did not immediately have to take their place – if she just gave the parents a bit of time they would work out a new balance for

---

*Doctors and therapists who prefer not to be so playful can quite properly ask the child to record the symptom systematically (e.g. time, location, duration, and strength) on a chart of his/her own making, for presentation at the next appointment. Implicitly or explicitly the patient is therefore being asked to keep the symptom going for the time being in order to help the doctor understand it better. I found this procedure remarkably effective with a 14-year-old severe asthmatic who still relied entirely on his mother to keep track of his attacks (in this case both of them were encouraged to keep a record), and I use it routinely, after a family interview, with children who soil themselves. They keep a daily record of their performances 'in pants', or 'in pan'. I make no attempt to encourage them one way or the other, as is common with star charts, which reward continence. The effect is to turn a regular disaster into a 'scientific experiment' which feels better for all the participants.

themselves, which would at least be good enough for her, if not for them. The little girl's idea of what changes are possible is far more conservative than her parents', so she blocks their development with her desperate solutions. But, as I say, this is the theoretical thinking behind this work, which helps me to think about families that are in transition. The family's actual experience will be quite different, and I do not necessarily get to know about it.

Conclusion

Although Groddeck seemed to understand it,[*] the idea of a psychological problem as a self-perpetuating function rather than a baffling and unnecessary irritant was developed as a clinical tool mainly in the United States by the very creative mixture of therapists, anthropologists and system-thinkers that congregated around Palo Alto in California in the 1950s, who gave birth to what is often known as Strategic therapy. Don Jackson[8] proposed the idea of prescribing the symptom and Jay Haley,[6] adapting the medical hypnotist Milton Erickson's techniques of sidestepping resistance, devised with his colleagues (including his wife Cloé Madanes) ways of re-defining the patient's activity so that it could no longer undermine the authority of parents and others trying to help. Several authors have written more recently about the application of these ideas to children with psychosomatic complaints, notably Michael White, an Australian family therapist who described getting children to practise having their symptoms to gain better control of them, and with the parents actively involved in these exercises.[18] Giving a name to a symptom is derived from another tradition, that of Gestalt therapy,[14] in which pain in particular can be relieved by encouraging the sufferer to accept it, through having to describe it in detail: the colour, location, shape, weight, size and so on. Both Strategic and Gestalt

---

[*]'It is possible to look upon every illness as a measure of protection against a worse fate' (op. cit., p. 210).

therapists have stressed that explanation is not much good without demonstration, so that therapeutic interventions tend to take the form of instructions to be put into practice, rather than simply as ideas to be thought about.

Witkin,[19] working in quite a different tradition, that of experimental psychology, provided some evidence that individuals with the classical psychosomatic diseases: ulcers, obesity, childhood asthma and diabetes, are over-involved and highly responsive to the people around them. So the idea of going beyond the individual to the intimate family group in the attempt to do psychotherapy with them makes sense, since the tension in the patient can be distributed around the family in a way that may be seen as helpful, but which is essentially unstable, so that the arrangement is bound to break down sooner or later, with a crisis resulting.

In support of this view I must mention Minuchin's major contributions to family treatment and research in psychosomatic medicine, for example his remarkable findings with the families of children with labile diabetes.[11] During a structured interview, in which the child watches the parents having a discussion, he measured the Free Fatty Acid levels (FFA) in the child and in the parents. The parents' Free Fatty Acid levels were raised when they got into an argument, but quickly fell when the child intervened. However, the child's intervention cost her a considerable rise in FFA levels, thus putting her at risk of diabetic symptoms. Furthermore, the FFA levels in the labile diabetic children did not return to normal during the recovery period, in contrast with other diabetics, thus leaving the child at risk for some time afterwards.

These findings suggest a physiological pathway through which sensitive children can respond to tensions in their parents, findings which are consistent with the ideas in this chapter; namely that, whether they like it or not, these children find themselves trying to rescue their parents when they seem to be in trouble. It is not known what mechanisms exist in children who are not diabetic, but it is clear that stress in childhood disease can be changed by intervening at a level which is outside the child's body yet can have effects within it.

References

1   Apley, J. and MacKlith, R. (1968), *The Child and his Symptoms: a comprehensive approach*, Oxford, Blackwell Scientific Publications (2nd edn).

2   Beautrais, A., Fergusson, D. and Shannon, F. (1982), 'Life Events and Childhood Morbidity: a prospective study', *Pediatrics*, vol. 70, no. 6, pp. 935-40.

3   Crossley, R. (1982), 'Hospital Admissions for Abdominal Pain in Childhood', *Journal of the Royal Society of Medicine*, vol. 75, pp. 772-6.

4   Elkan, J. (1977), 'Stages Towards the Containment of Mental Experience Illustrated in the Treatment of a Young Girl with Asthma', *Journal of Child Psychotherapy*, vol. 4 no. 3, pp. 90-105.

5   Groddeck, G. (1977), *The Meaning of Illness*, New York, International Universities Press.

6   Haley, J. (1973), *Uncommon Therapy: The psychiatric techniques of Milton H. Erickson, MD*, New York, W. W. Norton.

7   Hoffman, L. (1981), *Foundations of Family Therapy: A conceptual framework for systems change*, New York, Basic Books.

8   Jackson, D. (1963), 'A Suggestion for the Technical Handling of Paranoid Patients', *Psychiatry*, vol. 26, pp. 306-7.

9   Leaverton, D., White, C., McCormick, C., Smith, P. and Sheikholislam, B. (1980), 'Parental Loss Antecedent to Childhood Diabetes Mellitus', *Journal of the American Academy of Child Psychiatry*, vol. 19, pp. 678-89.

10 Madanes, C. (1980), 'Protection, Paradox, and Pretending', *Family Process*, vol. 19, no. 1, pp. 73-85.

11 Minuchin, S., Rosman, B. and Baker, L. (1978), *Psychosomatic Families: Anorexia Nervosa in Context*, Cambridge, Mass., Harvard University Press.

12 Nemiah, J. C., Freyberger, H. and Sifneos, P. E. (1976), 'Alexithymia: A View of the Psychosomatic Process', in *Modern Trends in Psychosomatic Medicine*, vol. 3 (ed. O. Hill), London, Butterworths.

13 Palazzoli, M. S., Boscolo, L., Cecchin, G. and Prata, G. (1978), *Paradox and Counterparadox: A new model in the therapy of the family in schizophrenic transaction*, New York, Jason Aronson.

14 Perls, F. S., Hefferline, R. F. and Goodman, P. (1973), *Gestalt Therapy: excitement and growth in the human personality*, Harmondsworth, Penguin Books.

15 Pickering, M. (1986), Letter to *The Guardian*, 27 June.
16 Searles, H. F. (1979), 'The Patient as Therapist to his Analyst', in *Countertransference and related subjects: selected papers*, New York, International Universities Press, pp. 380-459.
17 Walsh, F. W. (1978), 'Concurrent Grandparent Death and Birth of Schizophrenic Offspring: an Intriguing Finding', *Family Process*, vol. 17, no. 4, p. 457.
18 White, M. (1979), 'Structural and Strategic Approaches to Psychosomatic Families', *Family Process*, vol. 18, pp. 303-14.
19 Witkin, H. (1965), 'Psychological differentiation and forms of pathology', *Journal of Abnormal Psychology*, vol. 70, no. 5, pp. 317-36.

Health and illness in Chinese society

ROGER HILL

Roger Hill lives and practises acupuncture in Exeter. He is a Lecturer at the University of Exeter, where he is working towards establishing a Department of Complementary Health Studies. He is active in national complementary medical politics, and was involved in establishing the Council for Acupuncture and the Council for Complementary and Alternative Medicine. He is also active internationally, especially in opening up study exchanges with the People's Republic of China.

Chinese perspectives on 'health' and 'illness' are very different from our own: they are part of another world, with a philosophical tradition which mystifies as well as attracts us. Roger Hill offers here an overview of the way in which 'illness' is understood in China, from a personal as well as a social point of view.

The Chinese might be thought to have an obsession with health; it occupies a central place in their philosophy of life, and has stood them in good stead over the millennia. For the Chinese, health is more than the westerner's 'absence of disease', and more than the Japanese 'ability to recover quickly from whatever illness strikes'; it is clearly defined by positive physical, emotional and social characteristics.

Western doctors and others travelling with me on study tours in the People's Republic of China have commonly observed that the great majority of the population looks alert and healthy; 'there is no pathology on the streets', as one of

them put it. Despite earning only an average of US$?
capita per annum at the beginning of this decade,
placed them 138th in the world's income ratings, anc
the government having a mere US$10 per head to s
health care, the perinatal death rate – a good meas.....
nation's health – now stands among the best in the world, a
little better than the United Kingdom's at 1.3 per cent.

This situation is the result of a very successful recent public
health campaign. Yet this success itself is largely due to its
being based on a revival of ancient traditional concerns, which
were undermined only when the old order crumbled in the
first half of this century. The fabric of traditional society
dissolved, prompted by invasion from Japan, by predatorial
economic policy from Europe and the United States of
America, and by civil war within; and the country sank to an
uncharacteristic and desperate state of health.

A Canadian returning to China in 1970 after a thirty-year
absence was astounded by the obvious change and wrote:

> I searched for scurvy headed children, lice-ridden children,
> children with inflamed red eyes, children with bleeding
> gums, children with distended stomachs and spindly arms
> and legs. I looked for children covered with horrible sores
> on which flies feasted. I looked for children having a bowel
> movement, which, after much strain, would only eject
> tapeworms. I looked for child slaves in alley-way factories,
> children who worked twelve hours a day literally chained to
> press punches; children who if they lost a finger or worse
> were often cast into the streets to beg for future subsistence.

Instead, the author observed an astonishing picture of general
well being, almost unique in the world.

About a quarter of the world's population lives in the People's
Republic of China, and Chinese communities in other
countries (in Taiwan, Malaysia, Hong Kong, South East
Asia, North and South America, Europe) considerably augment

that number. No matter what their geographical location or political and economic background, they have in common certain beliefs and actions about health which unite them almost as much as the ideograms of their written language. Some informed Westerners suggest that this amounts to a blinkered ethnocentricity, and many ordinary observers still mutter in their minds about the mysterious orient, but the beliefs and actions are accessible to the outsider who is willing to explore a complex and ancient culture.

The Chinese are an extremely practical and down-to-earth race and base their ideas on a close observation of nature. Nonetheless it is also true that popular folk religion has its share of spirits, ghosts and devils and that much of the language of traditional psychiatric medicine is expressed in these terms. A study of Chinese literature shows how this nether world inhabits every corner of Chinese life.

Since the earliest references establishing Chinese culture, which stretch back to the first Emperor Fu Xi (c. 2852 BC) and his successor Shen Nong (c. 2780 BC), emphasis has been placed on the family, on the use of diet, herbs and other healing modalities, on exercise and on the systematic diagnosis of illness.

Emperors have played a pivotal part in the well-being of the Empire, standing as they did between Heaven and Earth. Their mandate to rule was confirmed (or otherwise) by all the signs and symptoms that befell their people; earthquakes, floods, good and bad harvests, comets and plagues were all heavenly portents and indicators of how well the Emperor was transmitting the heavenly influences to his people. In order to consolidate and point out the benefits of their rule, the Emperors instituted the tradition of state-sponsored scientific observation of all natural phenomena, which was conducted at the highest level.

Taoist precepts also encouraged the individual to a close study of nature with its qualities of unity and spontaneity. According to Taoism, it is man's duty to observe from a position that is free of preconceptions, to understand and to describe the observations, and by yielding to the flow of nature, to achieve the state of *wu wei*, 'actionless action'; the capacity to respond instantly to what is needed but to be free of desire to initiate action.

A passage in the *Tao-te-ching*, attributed to Lao-tse, reads:

Man is weak and pliant when he is born, solid and strong when he dies.
Herbs and trees are soft and lush when they germinate, parched and hard when they die.
For that which is solid and powerful is a part of death, that which is soft and weak is a part of life.
Therefore if the weapons are powerful, victory is impossible; a strong tree attracts the notice of the woodcutters.
Strength and power lie below; weakness and softness stand above.

By following nature, it was held that immortality could be achieved. Chinese religious life concentrates on making the most of what is here and now, rather than off-loading responsibility onto some elusive life to come. A lifestyle is adopted that conforms to natural law and emphasises its benefits. The Taoist 'Five Measures of Rice' sect (*c.* AD100) and others initiated various techniques designed to help achieve this. Two principal life-enhancing disciplines were used: inner ones comprising exercises such as *tai ji*, breathing exercises, *qi gong*, meditation and sexual restraint; and outer disciplines – proper nutrition leading to the use of herbs and medicines and the alchemical brewing of elixirs, though these last, despite nurturing some exciting proto-chemistry, backfired on the users as they turned more and more to heavy minerals of a decidedly toxic nature.

Immortality is scarcely the aim of most contemporary Chinese; rather, like the rest of us, they seek to avoid illness and make the most of the life they have, filling it out to give as much richness as is reasonable in the circumstances. The philosophy of 'making do with what is' is a fundamental Chinese characteristic, and it is one that saves them from much stress. Many of the ideas of ancient, esoteric Taoism, even so, are still found to be active, though muted, in everyday life throughout the Chinese world.

The great respect that is commonly shown for long life is represented in veneration of the elderly, and symbolically, in animals such as turtles (who have a long and slow life and who withdraw into their shells when life around them becomes inimical). The pine tree also symbolises long life and the capacity to stand firm and upright. It is frequently paired in paintings with the willow-tree representing softness, compliance, the ability to yield productively. Nature is commonly described thus in the pairing of opposites to generate a new and balanced whole, the coupling of *yin* and *yang*. The other great descriptive matrix is that of the five elements, or 'evolutive phases' as Porkert terms them in order to convey the idea that they are not descriptive of static slices of life but are ever-changing phases, ebbing and flowing. The five are wood, fire, earth, metal and water; each carries a chain of corresponding characteristics which through their intertwining convolutions reach out to the most subtle corners of life and provide a scale of reference for man as observer of nature and artefact. Contemporary doctors of traditional Chinese medicine of the highest sophistication still use the matrices of *yin* and *yang* and the five elements, evolved, enriched and amplified by centuries of case studies, in their diagnosis and treatment of patients. They do not deny the benefits of western science but prefer the use of their traditional language of life which thus aligns their treatments and advice with their patients' own language in describing every aspect of life – food, exercise, art, politics and social organisation.

The essential unit of Chinese society is the family. Maoism has done its best to weaken it in the People's Republic, but it survives despite thirty years of strident propaganda which has tried to teach that it is preferable to put the party (or state or commune or work unit) first. Elsewhere in the greater Chinese world, the strength of the family continues undiminished. The veneration of the family is one of the great legacies of

Confucianism that force in Chinese thought that balances out Taoism and Buddhism, as *yang* balances *yin* (both are necessary aspects of the human spirit, both are interdependent; neither can stand for long on its own). The notion and reality of the Chinese family embrace many minor arcana. The idea of continuity is enshrined in the respect for the family lineage, which reflects, albeit palely, the idea of immortality; the sense of reverence for elders, living and dead, echoes the idea of discipleship in the living faiths and arts. The family represents, to an individual, economic and social security, a safety-net in times of hardship and change. Family life, extended vertically and horizontally to the *n*th generation, is the warp and woof of the tapestry of society. From this the foreigner will almost always be excluded, hence his naive reaction of attributing inscrutability to an orient in which he has earned no part.

There are disadvantages too, for the individual. Studies such as those of the astute Linda Chih-ling Koo have shown that the emphasis that is placed on elder sons in particular to succeed in life can cause considerable stress. Similarly, youngest daughters, never highly valued in the Chinese social hierarchy, may be the butt-end of every family upset – there are no cats to kick nor much alcohol to take refuge in.

Because of this respect for the family, no shame may be brought upon it by having an unacceptable illness, in particular emotional and psychological ones. Thus there is a tendency to somatise stress into acceptable forms of ill-health (neurasthenia, nocturnal emissions, menstrual irregularities, etc.). Traditional Chinese medicine is neither deceived by this, nor does it need to change its therapeutic approach into a full-blooded western psychotherapy which would be totally unacceptable in Chinese culture. The wide-ranging correspondences of *yin* and *yang* and the five elements include subtle patterns of emotional dishar-monies that can be discussed and treated in the universal language of the Chinese mind without the shaming overtones that often accompany treatment by psychiatry. This idea of not treating separately matters of mind and spirit would be, I believe, of great value to Western cultures, where the incidence of neurosis is much higher than in oriental communities.

A distinction is made between *jian kang* (the condition of health) and *wei sheng* (the maintenance of health). The condition of health is reflected on four basic levels. The first is appearance; the way a person walks, the sound of his voice, his height and weight, smell, condition of tongue, colour of face, brightness of eye. Traditionally the body is treated with reverence, partly because it is valued in itself and partly for the sake of the family lineage. There was a time when surgery was shunned, but if it had to be done then the part of the body removed was kept to be buried eventually with the rest of the corpse. Punishments were tailored in severity to mutilate most those whose crimes were worst.

Sometimes this respect for the body is turned to scorn by western surgeons who wish to decry the way in which it was represented in traditional Chinese texts. But these were not based on limited observation of the human body or on insufficient knowledge of its workings (the circulation of the blood, for example, was described some ten centuries before Harvey) but, rather, medical knowledge was held to be so precious that it should only be taught to the initiated in a master-pupil relationship. Public representations were deliberately obscure, and certainly not to be taken at face value.

The idea of a microcosmic/macrocosmic relationship is common in Chinese thought. An analogy is frequently made between the earth's energy and that of man: the skeleton is compared to mountains, blood vessels to rivers. Earth's energy corresponds to the flow of 'qi' in man through the meridian system which is used in acupuncture. The practitioner of *feng-shui* – the geomancer who is responsible for harmonising man's energy to earth and by extension, to his artefacts on earth, buildings or graves – corresponds to the acupuncturist who is responsible for harmonising the *qi* or energy within man. Man's ideal role in nature resonates with each season, with each climate, with the place in which he lives and with the turn of every day. When the *qi* is in perfect balance, there is no place for disharmony or disease.

The second condition for health is the proper functioning of the internal organs - digestion, absorption, excretion, respiration and the miraculous working of nerves and fluids within the body. Their function and interdependence have long been acknowledged and carefully described, at least as far back as the *Huang Ti Nei Jing* (The Yellow Emperor's Classic of Internal Medicine) (c. 400 BC).

The discharges from the body, urine, excrement and so on, are carefully watched both by ordinary citizens and, more skilfully, by doctors for signs of disharmony. Traditional medicine demands the highest skills of phenomenology from its practitioners; the doctor is concerned with exactly how the patient is, through the direct experience of his own senses. No sign or symptom is unimportant – no shift of colour, no beat of the arterial pulse, no aspect of the nature of the illness itself – for the pattern of disharmony, described in the language of *yin* and *yang* and the five elements, is built up from the small clues presented by the patient. People suffer their illnesses in an individual way; the individuality needs to be fostered as much as the illness transformed.

The third condition of health rests on the belief that the emotions should not be allowed to fluctuate excessively, 'a soft temper is the root of a long life'. Peace of mind is held to be an essential pre-condition for good health, as is the fourth condition, which is social conformity.

Wei sheng, the art of health maintenance, is an obligation that is taken seriously by most Chinese people. The formidable achievements of the public health campaigns run in the People's Republic of China are an extension of a readily recognised private and family duty, and capitalise on it. Preventive medicine on both a self-help and a professional level has an honoured place in Chinese thinking.

In his book *Patients and Healers on the Context of Culture*, Arthur Kleinman lists the most common treatments used by families in Taiwan. Nutrition heads the table with 93 per cent of patients turning to dietary change in all cases of sickness; this is closely followed by the use of special foods and patent traditional medicines. Those of us brought up in the west with our impoverished taste of Chinese food being confined to the over-salted products of the local take-away, can have little idea of the richness of choice and subtlety of food demanded by the Chinese palate. Food is the first medicine; it too is classified by the *yin/yang* and five element criteria and is prescribed both to nourish and to harmonise the patient's *qi*. Western medicine is knowledgeable on how to nourish, but totally ignorant of how to harmonise the body's energies. It has no language for this.

Herbs and medicines are the extension of food. Although their applications have been carefully documented over 4000 years in China, there is an argument that their use is less desirable than other health maintenance measures. Paul Unschuld writes in *Medicine in China*:

> The belief in drugs as a valuable preventive and curative means releases man from a perceived necessity to follow a specific lifestyle as the basis of health. In the system of correspondence, this 'health' was defined as an integrated personal and social health. The one of these two aspects was guaranteed by the other, and both were maintained through a behaviour in conformity with a specific ethic. If personal health could be secured by means of drugs, the link with social health was severed and social order was no longer guaranteed because what better stimulus could be thought of to compel an individual to follow a strict code of moral norms than the reward of personal health! The concept of acupuncture differed from that of drug application in that it constantly reinforced the system of correspondences, providing stimuli only where man had not been able, owing to his own negligence or external conditions, to balance his existence in the proper way.

The public health campaigns in the People's Republic of China have reflected the traditional emphasis on personal and environmental hygiene. Onslaughts on the 'Four Pests' (rats, bedbugs, flies and mosquitoes), on cleaning the streets, on purifying water, on washing, on not spitting, all find their origins in the Xia dynasty (c. 2000 to 1500 BC). An excessively strong central government has the 'clout' to make these campaigns extremely effective.

Similarly, the People's Republic has continued the tradition of encouraging physical exercise. Throughout China, large numbers of people of all ages and conditions of health make their way to the city parks before dawn to practise the external exercises such as *tai ji* and *kung fu* and the internal ones such as *qi gong* and *nei gong*. But because of the communist reluctance to celebrate the particular character of the individual, some conflict has been experienced in allowing these disciplines which are based on Taoist ideas of *qi* and breath, and on Buddhist ones of meditation, calming the heart and purifying the spirit.

A healthy citizen in a communist state is one who is healthy enough merely to make an economic contribution to the nation, not one who goes beyond this to spend time celebrating his or her spiritual needs. But the spirit of man is irrepressible, and the need to realise it has ensured that Chinese people in all parts of the world transcend such difficulties. They continue to respect their refined and honourable traditions and to follow the precepts of *wei sheng*.

In the west the customary authoritarian relationship between doctor and patient is being challenged. Chinese ideas of illness, treatment, health and health maintenance may well play a useful role in informing and supporting this movement and in rebalancing a more productive partnership in the provision of our own health care.

7 · The meaning of illness: the homoeopathic approach

MISHA NORLAND

Misha Norland runs a homoeopathic practice and a school of homoeopathy in Devon, where he lives with his wife and four sons. He was born in Wales in 1943 of European refugees, and grew up in London. After leaving school, he was involved in a wide range of pursuits – from travelling to medical research, and from cleaning houses to directing films – before taking up homoeopathy fifteen years ago.

Classical homoeopathy, in both its understanding and treatment of illness, is radically different from allopathic medicine: it goes with, rather than opposes, disease. In this chapter, Misha Norland gives a basic explanation of homoeopathic theory and practice. He suggests as well how it may help us understand personal suffering, as well as collective afflictions such as cancer and AIDS.

For the homoeopath illness undoubtedly has meaning. Indeed, acquiring an understanding of the meaning of an illness should lead us, via the shortest route, to the cure. According to our understanding, the symptoms produced by the diseased organism are to be interpreted as an outward expression of internal disorder, a unique language, differing from case to case in subtle and vital ways. The symptoms provide the homoeopath with a true guide, leading towards the perception of what needs to be cured. We respect the 'voice' of the disease, the symptoms, as representing the best possible adaptation which the organism can muster in order to save

itself from a deeper, more permanent, more destructive form
of disturbance. Illness is a language making known and explicit
things which before had only been in the realm of implication,
things which have to be looked at, not buried like dirt under
the carpet, or in a routine way, removed with the surgeon's
knife.

It is common in depth psychology to think of disease, or
symptoms, as being a warning sign, a pointer for the
individual to alter the course of his or her life. In other words,
to take stock, to analyse and to redirect. This view is
contingent with the notion of psychosomatics in illness.
However, once a disease has established itself, and pathological
tissue changes have occurred, it is often very difficult, if not
impossible, for the individual to change sufficiently fast in
order for these changes to be reversed. It is at this point in
conventional medicine that patients subject themselves to
surgery, chemotherapy, radiation therapy, hormone replace-
ment therapy, etc. In an attempt to forestall the inevitable fate
that awaits them, the patient now views herself or himself as a
'victim', a victim of circumstances, a victim of Fate.

'I would rather be a pauper than a practitioner of medicine',
said Samuel Hahnemann, the founder of homoeopathy – for he
came to the belief (after a few years of medical practice) that it
was better to do nothing than to interfere with the lives of
patients using the heroic methods of his day. The orthodox
physician, past or present, basically wishes to name a disease
process. He has a sense of prognosis and armed with this,
together with a knowledge of how the disease may develop, he
suggests certain remedial measures. His training is such that he
tends to see the whole as no more than a sum of its parts;
looking at the human organism in a way that a plumber might
look at a heating system, in terms of pipes, pumps and vessels.
This arises out of a science which is based on the anatomy of
the corpse.

Now, the other approach to healing is to look at subtle
causes in relation to the whole being. A homoeopathic
physician would view the constitutional totality in descriptive

rather than causalistic terms; an analogical description of similarity between the patient and the remedy.

The word 'homoeopathy' implies the removal or annihilation of suffering by the administration of a like suffering; that likes shall be used to cure likes. As far as we know the first statement of this principle was by the Greek, Hippocrates; the second was by the alchemist, Paracelsus; and the third, was by Samuel Hahnemann, the founder of homoeopathy. In order to effect a cure by homoeopathic means, it is necessary to match the symptoms produced by the patient in disease, with symptoms that are produced by a medicinally active substance upon a healthy organism. Therefore, the study of homoeopathy involves the recording and analysis of disease symptoms and an understanding of the inner states, as well as the outer manifestations of medicinally active substances, the remedies. This latter process is known as 'proving'. Healthy volunteers, under the close observation of their physicians, take homoeo-pathically prepared substances until they experience a change in their normal state. These changes are recorded and the data thus obtained are collated and organised into a schema. The provings form the backbone of the *materia medica* of homoeo-pathic medicine.

I remember one of my teachers graphically describing how he proved Arsenicum upon himself in homoeopathic potencies. Being impatient, he wanted powerful effects so he really pushed the proving. He told how he ended up lying prostrate on the floor; he was vomiting and had diarrhoea; he was not able to reach up to the shelf for the antidote because he was so exhausted. He made the point that when you are proving, you should always have somebody in attendance to make sure they can get the antidote!

From the provings of Arsenicum we learn of internal burning, purging, diarrhoea, and prostration, coupled with tremendous anxiety. The provers fear that they will die, but the anxiety is not '...in any minute I will die' – it is rather a squirming, relentless anxiety that allows for no peace. It is this restlessness internally which expresses itself physically. They want to move but they do not have the energy to move – a terrible contradiction. For a brief spell the vital force is stronger than the poisoning force. Now the person will move position. They squirm and wriggle, then the force of the drug overwhelms them and they are prostrated. Also, because of the terrific draining of vitality, the person feels extremely cold, despite the feeling that they are burning inside. This character-istically gives rise to a desire for small sips of water, as though this might quench the internal fire. It is interesting to note that, at the deepest level, the restlessness and fear of Arsenicum expresses itself in terms of ontological uncertainty and terror of chaos to such a pathological degree that individuals who exhibit these characteristics are dependent, fearful of death and disease, terrified of disorder, and often have a compulsion to order everything in their environment – people as well as objects and concepts. For them disarray is intolerable.

I want to consider the question of why it should be that 'like cures like'. How can you extinguish fire with fire? It is not possible, obviously, to cure a burn by burning once again, because this would attack the organism at the level at which the disruption had occurred. In order to have an effect on the gross level you need to stimulate the subtle level. A remedy in a highly energised form, potentised and therefore capable of addressing itself to the formative, vital and healing energies in the organism would be selected according to the homoeo-pathic principle of similar action. In other words a substance capable of producing symptoms mirroring those of the action of fire would be selected and used as a stimulus.

When we are infected by, for instance, a flu virus, it may happen that we are overwhelmed because our defences are lowered. We experience symptoms: aching in our body, we feel bruised and shivery, our limbs are chilly and it is as though ice were placed upon our spine, we have no thirst, our head is hot and a dull and heavy pain suffuses our consciousness, we can hardly open our eyes, we want to be left alone. The symptoms are the response of the vital force to that morbific influence from outside; the best possible adaptation it can make. If we respond by taking aspirin, we counter that natural response, and the next day we may well be ill with sequelae. The wisest course would be to encourage the action of the vital force, allowing it to respond with a greater dynamism. We would, accordingly, prescribe the remedy known as Gelsemium, which in the provings is known to match these symptoms exactly.

We can perhaps understand more easily how a remedy can influence the operation of the vital force in such instances, by analogy with the laws of resonance. It is as though the remedy operated with the same characteristic frequencies as the disease-symptoms and thus, achieving resonance, amplifies its essential components.

It is said that Caruso could sing a note so powerfully that if he was in resonance with the wineglass on the table, the wineglass would shatter because the two frequencies were perfectly matched. Soldiers are told to break step when walking over a bridge because it has been observed that if they should march in step with a rhythm close to the resonant frequency of the bridge, the oscillations of the bridge might reach dangerous proportions.

When the frequency of the remedy is matched with the frequency of the disturbance very precisely, the amplitude is greatly increased. The organism, in its attempt to regain health throws off the disease by producing symptoms. The remedy helps the organism to intensify these symptoms, i.e. to throw off the disease more vigorously; and if this occurs, a cure should follow. Another observation arises from this model. For example, if the remedy is close but not perfect, we may still get an intensification and therefore a cure, but often the fact that there is an imperfection of match will produce symptoms which were not there before and which belong to the remedy given (i.e. spurious proving symptoms). The patient says 'My energy is better but now I have a few symptoms which I didn't have before.' You then explain that if they wait a while, the new transient symptoms will pass.

We inevitably encounter a rock against which the materialist mind shipwrecks itself and this is the question of potentised remedies. This was Hahnemann's brainchild. He wished to reduce the poisonous element in the medicine (some of the most potent remedies are very active poisons), while at the same time increasing their curative power.

If you were to dilute the medicine by putting one drop of it in a very large tankful of water and then administering a teaspoon of that substance to the patient, not very much would happen. However, when diluted in successive stages by one drop to 99 drops, whilst at every stage subjecting the dilutions to mechanical energy – a process known as succussion, or, in the case of insoluble substances, grinding them in a pestle and mortar – this has a very surprising effect. It does exactly what Hahnemann had intended: it increases the medicinal activity while reducing the quantity of the physical remedy-substance administered. This process is repeated successively: at each stage the substance acquires greater potency. Soon we have dilutions of one in a billion, or one in a trillion, and we pass a point where there is indeed a very small probability of even having one molecule of the medicinal substance present in the dilution. But, and this is the nub, the potency increases.

We may think of this in terms of a continuum between the spiritual pole, on the one hand, and the physical world with all manifest things, on the other. When we potentise a remedy we are spiritualising it. Sickness is a psychophysical effect of a disturbance of the spiritual vital force.[*] The homoeopathic

[*] 9 *Vital Force* In the healthy condition of man, the spiritual vital force (autocracy), the dynamis that animates the material body (organism), rules with unbounded sway, and retains all the parts of the organism in admirable, harmonious, vital operation, as regards both sensations and functions, so that our indwelling, reason-gifted

prescriber matches the symptoms produced by the provings of a remedy, with the symptoms produced in the sick person; in order to heal we need to go to the spiritual pole and thus we use potentised remedies in order to reach the source of the disturbance and to effect change.

When the simillimum is administered to a sick person, the first thing that is experienced is an increased sense of well-being; an increase of energy. Following this the patient usually experiences a temporary intensification of presenting symptoms. Then, as the reversal of the disease process takes place, there is a quite characteristic movement. This movement has been plotted by the homoeopath Constantine Hering and is often called simply Hering's Law, or the Law of Cure. According to this law the direction of cure is from within to without; from more important organs to less important and more peripheral organs; from above to below; and in reverse direction so that the last symptom to appear will be the first to be cured and the first symptom to have appeared will be the last to be cured. In fact 'from above to below' – is not always strictly true. Though it gives the idea of general direction, sometimes the shortest route from an important organ to a less important organ may not be 'from above to below'. The centrifugal aspect of cure, however, is fundamental to Hering's Law.

This idea of a direction of movement – from within to without – brings us to the notion of hierarchies, because we

mind can freely employ this living, healthy instrument for the higher purposes of our existence.
10   The material organism, without the vital force, is capable of no sensation, no function, no self preservation; †it derives all sensation and performs all the functions of life solely by means of the immaterial being (the vital principle) which animates the material organism in health and in disease.

† 'It is dead, and now only subject to the power of the external physical world; it decays, and is again resolved into its chemical constituents.'
(Aphorisms 9 and 10, *Organon of Medicine*, Samuel Hahnemann, Ed. V.)

could ask 'What is within?' For instance, after prescribing for a claustrophobic patient, they develop a terrific spasm of sobbing and feel that they have a lump in the throat. They think they are worse. Before they could not go out at all, but now they have an emotional crisis which reminds them of the great trauma of grief ten years ago when their partner died. The homoeopath is delighted because a release has occurred: the claustrophobia was the best possible option for that person's psyche given that the grief had been suppressed. Once the grief has been released some minor physical symptoms may appear. Perhaps now they will develop a little eczema, such as they also had in their teens around the time of their first love disappointments. We see the symptoms returning in reverse order of their appearance, during 'cure'.

Let us look again at the chronology of events. The first grief was exteriorised, but the eczema had been suppressed with creams. The second grief, being built upon the incomplete adaptation to the original grief, instead of resulting in a flood of tears, was 'bitten back'. And as a result of this suppression the patient has developed fears and phobias. There are many possible outcomes, many ways in which the psyche can respond. Fears and phobias are one possible outcome, but another could, for example, be a neurological disorder, such as paralysis.

Sometimes things do not work out quite so clearly. Somebody who has a very serious disorder, like cancer, has very likely suppressed the emotional level so effectively that the whole disease-force has been encapsulated into this mass of degenerating tissue. You can see why the surgeon wants to cut it out. During the process of cure we may find that there will be a release in the emotional realm. For instance, suddenly there will be great anger and resentment, for when the level of pathology is great, its emotional analogue is also great. To give another example: people who have multiple sclerosis, especially in advanced stages, are often emotionally very serene and mentally in a state of euphoric clarity. During the process of cure this level of serenity and clarity may be temporarily

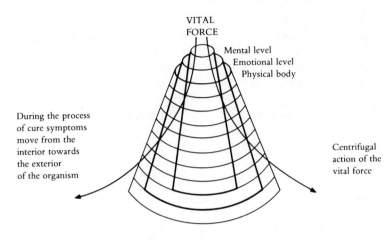

VITAL
FORCE

Mental level
Emotional level
Physical body

During the process
of cure symptoms
move from the
interior towards
the exterior
of the organism

Centrifugal
action of the
vital force

Fig.1

erased and replaced by hopelessness and despair, which is the
mental/emotional equivalent of the neurological disorder.

Fig.1 is a schema from the homoeopath, George Vithoulkas. It
shows three cones, one within the other. The central and
highest cone represents the mental realm, the next the
emotional, and the outside and lowest cone represents the
physical body.

Let us look at the physical part of the hierarchy, relating to
the relative importance of organs. The most important organs,
without which we would be instantly dead, are the brain and
heart. These correspond symbolically to the two functions of
thinking and feeling respectively. These we place at the top of
the hierarchy. At the bottom of the hierarchy we find the skin
– the envelope. Between these are, respectively, the nervous
system (and this includes both central and autonomic nervous
systems), the endocrine system, kidneys, liver, lungs, the
stomach, bones and muscles.

There are certain characteristic examples of Hering's Law of

Cure which we meet time and time again, e.g. asthma in the process of cure disappears and skin eruptions come out. Or in the case of heart disease, the person develops the rheumatic symptoms that they had prior to the onset of heart trouble. Generally speaking, we find that one of the reasons that disease has moved inwards is due to suppression. (Another is due to the natural diminution of the vital force through aging leading to a decrease in the centrifugal action of vitality.) The child has eczema, the parent takes the child to the doctor and suppressive ointment is put on. If the vitality of the child is not strong (because of constitutional weakness) then the skin symptoms will disappear. Some years later and apparently unconnected, say at a time when the child is under stress at school coming up to the examination period, she develops asthma. Likely as not the asthma will be suppressed, and a nervous condition may develop. Now the child develops a state of great anxiety with a series of emotional problems including fears. In this example we can see the development of disease from the skin, at the bottom of the hierarchy, to lungs, through to fears and emotional disturbances.

The hierarchy of the emotional aspect of mankind is, because of its fluidic nature, the most difficult to plot. However, roughly speaking, we may see suicidal disposition (lack of love of self) and sustained rage (lack of love of others) as two sides of the most profound disturbance of the emotional hierarchy. This may be followed by apathy and indifference. Then we might arrange a descending scale of pathology thus: anguish, fears and phobias, sadness, dissatisfaction, irritability.

Let us sketch the hierarchy of the mind, the will and understanding. Understanding belongs to statements like 'I am', or 'I know who I am.' The moment I start losing that sense of my own identity, I am afflicted by the deepest level of sickness. This is followed by paranoid ideas, delusions, hallucinations, dullness and loss of the power to reason. Lower yet, we have memory, which we can sub-divide into long- and short-term. In the provings we find that certain remedies interfere with the ability to reason or with memory, some

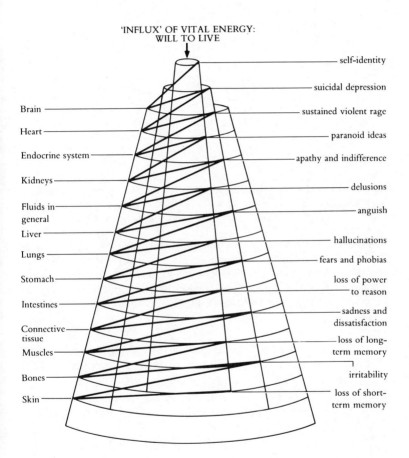

'INFLUX' OF VITAL ENERGY:
WILL TO LIVE

self-identity

suicidal depression

Brain — sustained violent rage

Heart — paranoid ideas

Endocrine system — apathy and indifference

Kidneys — delusions

Fluids in general — anguish

Liver — hallucinations

Lungs — fears and phobias

Stomach — loss of power to reason

Intestines — sadness and dissatisfaction

Connective tissue — loss of long-term memory

Muscles — irritability

Bones — loss of short-term memory

Skin

Fig.2

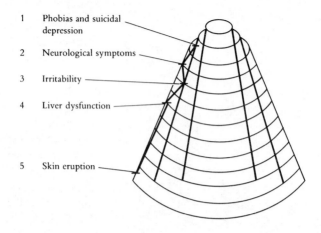

1 Phobias and suicidal depression

2 Neurological symptoms

3 Irritability

4 Liver dysfunction

5 Skin eruption

Fig. 3 Illustration of the change in centre of gravity in a case involving alternating correspondences of emotional and physical levels. At point 1, the patient presents the prescriber with a totality of symptoms with centre of gravity on the emotional level. After treatment, the centre of gravity moves to the physical level at point 2. With further treatment the centre of gravity again shifts back to the emotional level, point 3, but at a lower level of correspondence. Then, as treatment progresses, the centre of gravity again moves peripherally to point 4 and finally point 5 before the patient is fully cured.

produce hallucinations, some even interfere with our sense of identity. Some remedies so interfere with a person's internal organisation that they cease to want to live. For them everything is black and nothing so desirable as the very thought of suicide, which like sweet music makes them feel at peace.

There is but one disturbance in the vital force and it manifests itself through the various outlets that are available to it at any given time; at one time it manifests itself in the skin, at another time in the lungs, and at yet another time it will manifest with fears and phobias.

What is the nature of the energies that manifest as pathological signs in mind, emotions and body? And where do they come from? I would like to address these questions with a metaphor: Imagine a seed. This seed represents the potential of the individual. It grows in the womb of the soil, nurtured by water and the warmth of the sun. And given the conditions of spring – warmth and water – it begins to germinate and make its growth towards the sun. We can imagine here a polarity between Heaven and Earth, a vertical relationship between the material world, and the spiritual world to which all things aspire in their growth; aspiring to express what is in the inner kernel of their being. There is likely to be a point, maybe quite early on in the experience of the organism, where some stress occurs; some block occludes for the time being the rays of the sun. Now the organism is required to adapt. It has to make a movement around the obstacle in order to carry on its journey towards the sun. It is at this point, the point of adaptation to stress, that symptoms may be produced. These arise as a consequence of the interaction between the stress factor and the individual character of the organism.

Continuing with the metaphor, let us picture a sunflower. Imagine that you can see the flower (the emotional symptoms), and now the leaves (the physical symptoms). And then you recognise the seeds as those of the sunflower (the mental symptoms). The flower, leaves and seeds are all parts of the sunflower, but at different phases of development. A botanist will recognise these as different parts as well as stages in the life of the plant. In like manner the homoeopath will recognise the different stages of disease as belonging to one central theme. The homoeopathic prescriber's task is to find and administer the simillimum.

I do not wish to give the impression that all a person ever needs is their one constitutional remedy, representing the constitutional totality of the patient; that golden thread which runs through the patient from the first until the last. It is like unravelling a ball of string. You have to undo the ball and take out all the knots; you have to experience all that has happened, in order to be able to put it back together in a more coherent and harmonious way. Or, to use another image, it is like stripping the layers of an onion, one by one.

When prescribing you have an idea of what is going on in the centre, of what the seed kernel is like, yet people nevertheless express themselves according to the way they are now. Thus the homoeopathic prescription is aimed at dealing with whatever is happening in time present. When we re-take the case after a suitable time lapse, what we may observe is the layer below, now expressing itself in time present. We prescribe according to that picture.

Sometimes it happens that the inner penetrates right through to the outside. When inner and outer meet the way is clear to prescribe the one (constitutional) remedy which will raise the person's vital energy to such a high degree that they are then able to break the bonds of disease, the old ties which bind them in the strangle-hold of inappropriate behavioural patterns.

At the origin, the source of all things, there is formless potential. And arising out of this there stream forth the energy forms of all things which eventually will become manifest as the shapes and patterns of the material universe. It is as though there are rays, streams of continuous creation between the formless energy on the one hand and the created universe on the other.

Basically, there are two models that are drawn by homoeopaths. One states that there is one single connection from spirit right down to matter. This is described as a ray. This represents the whole of the suffering we experience, the disfigurement of the vital force in its entirety. It also constitutes the *one* remedy – for the sake of illustration, we shall name it Sulphur. Another model states that Sulphur played this role for a time, but that the situation then changed; the ray branched off to another remedy.

A homoeopathic practitioner prescribes on the basis of what is closest to the pole of matter; in other words, that which is revealed to him or her at the time of the consultation. To the extent that the stimulus of the remedy is able to push the vital force into release, symptoms will successively appear, demonstrating Hering's Law of Cure.

There are some fundamental remedies which come into play at the beginning of life, the greatest polycrests. Polycrest remedies are those which in the provings affect every part of the human economy. They are therefore part of the common experience, and remedies used often in everyday practice. Hahnemann suggests that there are three fundamental remedies around which the others may be grouped. Sulphur, Calcarea Carbonicum and Lycopodium.

Since Sulphur exists in matter *and* as an energy or thought form, we can picture the energy of Sulphur streaming down from the pole of spirit to the material level where it manifests as the element. When we say that we are sick and manifesting symptoms of Sulphur, what we mean is that this ray of energy is broken and we are suffering a disconnection. It is because of this particular disconnection that we are producing the symptoms of Sulphur: 'itching skin eruptions, burning pains, 11 a.m. aggravation, thirst for cold water, fear and vertigo when in high places, indolence, a mind which is very active, theorising, but doesn't wish to bring anything into actuality'. It is precisely at the point of disconnection that symptoms begin to manifest. When we potentise the element Sulphur, the process raises the remedy-substance towards the pole of spirit and it becomes effective as a curative agent capable of rejoining the patient with the spiritual ray of Sulphur.

In the healthy person all the energies stream through like the kaleidoscopically changing colours of a moving crystal. Of every energy we are a channel. It is when those channels of energy are blocked that we become sick. The blockages occur for very many reasons, some of which are inherited, some karmic, and some due to our inability to adapt to stresses. All of these inter-relate, of course, and even if we cannot see the weaver, yet with careful observation, recording and study we can become aware of the pattern being woven.

The living organism is in a state of dynamic balance. It is constantly adjusting itself to changes within the environment. It is like a dance between partners except that in this dance there are very many partners. A dance of continual movement and interaction, in which the vital force makes adjustments constantly to keep the organism within a state of dynamic equilibrium.

The way in which we react to stresses, accidents, infection and so on, is very much determined by our disposition. For example, if I am involved in a brawl and am hit, the resulting disequilibrium and shock may well pass quickly with no longer-term damage. On the other hand, I may be overwhelmed, the state of shock freezing me, as it were, in that moment. Should this non-adaptation continue, it could result in various forms of pathology.

And in an even deeper way it seems that not only the way in which agents of disease and stress affect us, but also the events life brings us, are in some deep way intrinsic to us. Though the stimulus or event appears to come at us from outside, there is a deep correspondence between what happens in the outer world and our unique disposition. The events in our lives are an expression of our inner selves; even a so called accident may often, in retrospect, be understood to be the outward expression of an inner imperative. And the remedy chosen after the 'accident' and prescribed because of the accident reconnects the 'victim' with his, or her source, thus eliminating the need for further exteriorisations.

Life affects us and moves us in a way which is characteristic, like a gnarled old tree that has withstood the blasting gales of experience. It may be a magnificent tree. I am not suggesting the remedy ungnarls you but it allows energy access to every part – so that you can be gnarled and magnificent.

Hahnemann, in the ninth Aphorism of his Organon, talks about the 'dynamis', the vital force that animates and coordinates the physical body. He says that our purpose is to allow 'our indwelling, reason-gifted mind...to freely employ this living healthy instrument for the highest purposes of existence.' And it is this issue of what is meant by 'the higher purposes of existence', which is germane. Homoeopathic treatment attempts to free us, to express our unique individuality, and to reach towards our greatest potential, so that we might grow towards the Spiritual Sun, and our true inheritance. The question is: how is that to be achieved?

I believe that 'aggravation before cure' is a necessary part of the process. In order to experience release from suffering, one has first of all to intensify suffering. A growth curve moves in this manner: there is a fall, maybe even to the very darkest depths of despair. The darkness is only transitory and there comes a point where the light is seen again, and one begins an upward journey. The way up is usually harder than the fall, but the whole process of having fallen and having seen light at this moment of greatest despair means that one's individual strength and energy is greater and vitality increases. After a period of grace, one usually moves into a period of stagnation, where one feels that things are good, but there is no further development. We may then experience a slight drop in energy.

To reach upwards towards the new, the inventive, the creative one has to descend once again into the pool of potentiality, that atavistic movement into simple suffering, the past (both personal, hereditary and collective) which contains the ungerminated seeds waiting their turn to be activated. The seeds of suffering are released homoeopathically from suffering by suffering.

Appendix 1 – AIDS

While holding with the belief that collective phenomena such
as epidemic diseases should be tackled in the individual
suffering the disease, I nevertheless feel that a few words about
the collective would be in order. After all, the laudification of
the individual ego, as apart from the group, is a relatively
recent occurrence. In our culture we may relate it to the
diminution of the power of the church and the monarchy. Just
before this shift of emphasis and heralding it by a few hundred
years, we witnessed the plague in Europe, and the spread of
syphilis.

We now stand at the threshold of a new scourge, AIDS,
faced with the burning question of how to behave; especially in
view of the fact that despite our great technological ingenuity
we have as yet no 'cure'. We cannot command chastity,
enforce monogamy, outlaw adolescent experimentation, without radical reform. We cannot simultaneously uphold the
rights of the individual and free enterprise whilst enforcing
totalitarianism; or put the group needs before that of the
individual, as happens in war when government recruits
individuals to fight for the survival of the group. Yet this is, I
believe a closely analogous situation to the one in which we
find ourselves. I would not, however, propose a political
solution; for government, with its structures for law and
enforcement, could not successfully deal with the problems of
contagion, even if such measures were deemed desirable.

A plague cannot be dealt with as though it were a criminal,
or an aggressive neighbouring state. The very word 'plague'
conjures up such potent images from the past that we hardly
dare use it. Yet AIDS is just such a phenomenon. A plague
may be described as a potent destructive force affecting large
portions of the community without regard to profession, creed
or colour. Furthermore, it is not amenable to cure by the
methods available at the time. It may be a fact that, as one
American doctor put it, AIDS was incubated in the brothels of
Africa and the homosexual clubs of New York, yet its effects

are becoming widespread. The fact that we instinctively wish to push responsibility, the shadow side of our nature, into the darkness, does not diminish our susceptibility to the disease, indeed it may enhance it. It is all too easy to identify a scapegoat 'out there' rather than to look within at the roots of suffering. It has been said that each age acquires the disease which it has earned and which is uniquely expressive of its inner conflicts.

Born out of our recent history of conflicts and wars, we see a society steeped in a noxious mixture of fear and violence. The physical counterpart of this manifests as diseases of ever-increasing morbidity. The invisible element in this unhappy scenario is the element of suppression. Suppression may be seen to be an arch villain in the piece, for without it the natural inclination of the organism would be to exteriorise disease. Like any effective villain, suppression dons a multitude of guises, the most odious of which (like the road to Hell which is paved with good intentions) wears the costume of medical researcher, pharmaceutical manufacturer and prescriber of drugs, and doctor. It is nothing short of tragic to note that by these means (and good intentions) the health of the nation is undermined.

Whatever AIDS may represent collectively, karmically, miasmatically, or in terms of the sick individual, we shall most probably agree that good health offers the best chance for survival. AIDS (acquired immunity deficiency syndrome) is without doubt the most inward of epidemic contagious diseases to date, not merely because it is transmitted sexually and by the blood, but also because it directly affects the immune defence system leaving the organism defenceless. We may speculate upon the mechanism of this occurrence. George Vithoulkas suggests that the repeated use of antibiotics in cases of recurring venereal contagion progressively undermines the immune system until it eventually breaks down, to which we may add another factor, immunisation. Repeated immunisations, especially of infants, since it operates by warning the immune system and keeping it on red-alert, puts great strain upon the organism (as if it had actually engaged in battle but without the resultant resolution, i.e. death or recovery). Although the *modus operandi* of inoculation is homoeopathic, the method is gross, for disease products (however modified) are actually introduced into the blood-stream (with the exception of oral polio).

The 'virus' of the inoculation, being denatured, initiates the production of antibodies without overwhelming the organism with symptoms of the gross disease. It is precisely because of this non-production of symptoms that the greatest danger results.

Let us examine various options from the point of view of vital reaction: We can define four basic categories; these I have arranged in chronological order of increasing pathology. The first group comprises those individuals in whom the vital force is strong and who have a good hereditary background. These individuals will experience an acute episode characterised by fever and mild malaise; this being the organism's successful exteriorisation of the effects of the inoculation. The individuals will not be plagued by sequelae. The second group differs from the first in having a temporarily weakened vitality while yet having good heredity. This weakness may be due to such factors as poor nutrition, lack of adequate sanitation, emotional deprivation, or cruelty. Because of lowered vitality the body's reaction is sluggish, the fever slow to develop, and may be of a low-grade, malignant type which is only gradually resolved. However, once resolved no constitutional weaknesses remain. The third group comprises those who have a poor heredity (i.e. they are miasmatically* loaded), yet they do possess a strong vitality. These individuals respond with rapidity, but

---

Miasm: sins of our forefathers visited upon future generations – specifically the hereditary stigma of disease, named by Hahnemann as Psora (the itch), Sycosis (catarrh, rheumatism and neoplasms), Syphilis (destructive tendencies, necrosis), to which some homoeopaths add the constitutional and hereditary effects of tuberculosis and cancer and to which AIDS will no doubt be added in the future.

the effects of the inoculation linger on in the form of constitutional troubles dating back to the time of immunisation. The fourth group comprises those who have a weak vitality and also poor heredity. Those in this group experience no reaction, no fever, the effects of the inoculation strike inwards producing either deep and often neurological pathologies such as paralysis, mental and behavioural disturbances, or such slowly developing symptoms as elude short-term detection. Certain members of these last two groups are recognised as being at risk and are therefore not immunised. Despite this, babies of tubercular parents are protected with 'BCG', and the more remote hereditary background not taken into account as though all the work upon inheritance had never been carried out.

Why do we inoculate? Clearly it is in the belief that by so doing we may avert a danger that the future may hold. Perhaps fear makes fools of us all? Do we not note the concomitant increase in chronic disease with the removal of epidemics? While reducing infant mortality, are we possibly increasing adult suffering?

The hope of homoeopaths is that this method (i.e. homoeopathy) be used to treat diseases as and when they occur so that the individuals thus fortified by successful adaptation to experience may grow up without the handicaps which are so often the results of medical practice and also with a lessened miasmatic load. An individual who is enabled to work out, exteriorise and thus illuminate inner suffering will not only be free from unnatural drives, but also will parent healthier and happier children. Thus, collective phenomena may be influenced by the efforts of individuals.

I have not addressed the question of our karmic inheritance and the shift in consciousness heralded by AIDS since it is so speculative in character. From a materialistic standpoint we note that, as a consequence of the venereal nature of the contagion, monogamy is the safest method of remaining uninfected. This may lead us to speculate about the cyclic nature of sexual repression and freedom, to note that the swing away from Victorian moral attitudes has lead to an overcompensation in the form of a relaxed moral stance in which the cornerstones of our social structure are being undermined: the institution of marriage, traditional labour relations, social services, etc. In the place of these we witness great social unrest set against the backdrop of the arms race, terrorism, rape, drug abuse, etc. As I have suggested, AIDS may be viewed as a materialisation of these trends – the best possible adaptation by the vital force of the collective unconsciousness of the race. It protects the collective organism from possibly even more destructive pathology. Perhaps a nuclear holocaust, or the consequences of pollution, deforestation or other eco-catastrophes. (It was T. S. Eliot who suggested in his *The Wasteland* that the world might end with a whimper.) Planetary self-regulation working as it does for the survival of the whole organism is impartial as to which isolated individual falls prey to whatever disease, call it plague, or fate, that may be currently manifesting. However, by applying the ancient doctrine of 'microcosm like unto macrocosm' we would expect the body of the planet to regulate itself in a homoeostatic manner and also follow a centrifugal mode of elimination during the process of cure. Furthermore we would expect to witness an intensification of presenting symptoms (an aggravation) prior to elimination, resolution and cure.

It seems to me that we are still heading towards aggravation and it is my hope that the pressure is sufficient to herald a radical change, for radical it must indeed be.

Viewed with optimism such phenomena as the rise of interest in meditation and awareness-raising techniques, alternative and complementary medicine, ecology and feminism, whilst being taken to extremes by some, may herald a new way. The Aquarian age is symbolised by the water carrier; man carrying a pitcher of water, associated, according to Jung, with the function of feeling, by others with brotherhood and co-operation, and ruled by the planets Uranus and Saturn. Uranus is associated with renovation and revolution, Saturn with restriction and realisation. It is interesting to consider the significance of these symbols in relation to the collective themes of our time.

Appendix 2

Karma is the law of action and reaction played out upon the stages of many reincarnations.

So universal is this law, call it fate or fortune, that we must concede that all events, however trivial, are the result of karma.

We may distinguish two grades of karmic influence:

(1) such action as has been initiated or ended during this lifetime; those actions over which we may exercise a degree of free will;

(2) that which we have created during our past lives and which now exerts influence over us through essentially subconscious and soul processes, also through collective and racial traits.

In the Christian tradition we may therefore speak of free will in relation to the first category and fate in relation to the second.

All events are the results of karmic, soul processes. For this perspective illness, accidents and all forms of suffering are the results of past actions, unprocessed soul residues. At the moment of death of the body we experience a division and separation of light and dark elements (spirit, and earth bound soul elements) the first of which, being light and airy, soars up and leaves the heavier earthy matter below. The dense matter holds within its gravitational field all life's experiences. So identified with this life are we that we call this 'reality' and fear its passing. So greatly do we cling to these memories and residues of our former life and lives that this soul stuff forms the connection, and the gravitational field within which our next incarnation may manifest.

C. G. Jung (who does not openly speak of karma) states that the psyche may be pictured as consisting of the smaller illuminated area of consciousness floating above, as it were, the dark sea of infinite possibilities, the subconscious. Arising out of the subconscious are the motive and frequently instinctual drives which determine our lives. The process of individuation and growth may be seen as a conscious awakening and therefore as casting light upon our subconscious drives; creating a pathway between spirit and soul, so that the body may be employed by the spirit for the higher purposes of our existence.

That which Jung calls the shadow, the area of darkness into which we cast all those parts of ourselves of which we do not approve, when no longer denied and reviled offers up great sources of energy which had hitherto been tied up in the knot of self-denial and self-hatred. Both physical and mental illness may be understood to be expressions of these repressed drives; these are the results of the first category of karmic activity over which we may exercise free will. The second category of karmic influence is manifest in such phenomena as hereditary disease, uterine trauma, birth trauma and childhood fatalities. The genius and the cretin, the athlete and the spastic have each chosen this incarnation of suffering and rejoicing, to uniquely express their individual journey of learning and discovery.

Karmic influence extends to include all things, not only the diseases we are heir to and the style of healing we adopt to reverse degenerative processes, but also the race as a whole. By way of example we may cite the race of the Jewish slaves who escaped from mighty Egypt. Born of great suffering, theirs was the first monotheistic religion; out of the blood and earth of oppression arose a people who believed that theirs was the only true God. A clever race who often spoke three languages: the common tongue of the people of the land they inhabited; their own common language, Yiddish; and the sacred language, Hebrew. Small wonder then that jealousy and hatred should dog their passage through history culminating in the great purge, the 'final solution', of the Third Reich. Here, too, the German nation after continual scrapping with neighbouring states felt itself to be small, oppressed and inferior, and arising out of the blood and earth (a Nazi slogan)*of oppression, they

---

Blood and earth: the sacrifice. The victim's blood, the heat of life, the spiritual aspect of the organism is re-united with earth in sacrifice,

almost succeeded in their endeavours to exterminate the Jews and create the great empire of the Aryan races. And now the Jews in Israel find themselves still at war, continually at war, a chronic unhealing ulcer, a sore spot upon the face of the earth. This example illustrates the notion of racial karma.

Looking at the earth as a whole, we cannot fail to see a suffering entity with localised regions of particular disturbance; the vents through which the poison within is expelled. Through healing the individual and thus enabling disease forces an outlet we may hope to reduce the influence of karma leading to the eventual healing of the totality within which we live: the race and the environment.

Footnote continued from page 107

where one is butchered to purify the tribe, or the tribe to purify the nation. The Jews called this the holocaust after the ritual practised in ancient Greece, where the sacrificial beast was burnt, holocausted, just as they had been in the ovens of Auschwitz and Buchenwald.

8 · The patient as healer: how we can take part in our own recovery

PAT KITTO

Pat Kitto is a private counsellor working with cancer patients and others. She uses various approaches, including transpersonal psychology, gestalt, message and healing. Her main interest is in relaxation/meditation techniques using visualisation and healing. She runs workshops and works part-time with the Bristol Cancer Help Centre.

Pat Kitto is highly committed to the practice of self-healing, and her contribution is based on years of practical experience in enabling people to become involved in the treatment of their illnesses. She founded and worked for many years with the Totnes Natural Health Centre.

She said: 'Until I had cancer I never knew what it was to be ill. I didn't know what it was to rely on others. I had never experienced that terrible panic you get when you're told you have cancer. Now that I have experienced it, I can honestly say that I wouldn't have been without it.'

Later she explained why. It had to do with getting close to an entirely different side of herself. She felt as though she had touched something important in her own personality, the person she had lived with all her life and never really met.

'I used to race through life at sixty miles an hour,' she said. 'I never thought of caring for myself. I liked a drink with the

109

girls, working hard, a giggly evening in the pub. I never thought of being quiet for more than two minutes at a time. And look at me now, meditating! And really enjoying silence and even finding time to read and paint. It's like another world. Being able to talk to people about real things and finding I can help them. I wouldn't ever have believed it was possible!'

Most of us are ill at some time in our lives. Some of us spend many months, even years being unwell. Could it be that there is something for us to learn through these experiences? Until I worked with cancer patients and other ill people, I would never have expected them to express gratitude for being ill. But many do.

Even so, what right have we, who are apparently fit and well, to talk about *the meaning of illness* to people who are ill or close to those who are suffering? It can sound hard, even irrelevant. Pain and invasive forms of illness have, in the last analysis, to be dealt with by the person concerned. Whatever support the ill person receives from doctor, hospital, family or friends, only he or she can know the quality and depth of that suffering. To suppose that anyone can evaluate their state in terms of 'meaning' might seem totally inhuman.

Yet for every one of us who believes in the importance of wholeness in our personalities, and I am certainly one, there has to be an awareness of the dark as well as the light side of life. Without both of these there would be no real humanity to our existence. This acceptance of the whole means that suffering, dispair, illness and death are as much part of us as love, joy, exploration and occasional ecstasy. It is the way in which we react to these two sides of ourselves which makes us learn and grow and ultimately learn how to respect and appreciate life.

When we consider the meaning of illness, we have to ask questions about the emotional, mental and spiritual parts of ourselves as well as the physical. We are more than just a body with physical needs. When sickness comes, even in the shape of a broken arm, it comes to the whole person. And in the struggle to adjust, it may dominate everything and everyone around us.

Illness is something which affects the smooth working of our lives. It stops our work patterns, interferes with our relationships, allows pain or distress to invade us, and stops us from pursuing our dreams. It can be anything from a slight fever to a devastating illness like multiple sclerosis. Even the slightest deviation from what we think of as health can have a traumatic effect. We assume that health requires that we are in balance and in control. As we all yearn to be in control, the sense of loss we experience when we become ill can be very acute.

However, we begin to learn that what appears to be health in a person is often not true balance but a state of desperate fragility kept in control by suppression of real needs. Many people have no real sense of self-worth or are unable to express such emotions as anger, hate or love. We live in a society which nurtures the intellect at the expense of other forms of expression. A child learns early that emotional behaviour does not earn him or her the respect of parents. When we become ill there is often the overwhelming realisation, and relief, that we can show emotion. It dramatically changes the scene, and opens up new and different ways of being and relating, which were not acceptable to us when we were 'healthy'.

Illness can mean different things to different people. For some it can be something inexplicable, dark and draining: experienced as total isolation from the apparently healthy people around. For others it can be a valuable time to withdraw from life, to reassess, to make some change in life or attitudes. For any individual, the area of life which is touched by illness may be quite personal. Here I shall just mention some rather common experiences:

- • We may realise that we need love, touch and attention from others. Many of us do not discover real feelings of love until we are ill. We may pretend that we do not need love in our lives, or conclude that because we find relationships difficult it is better to keep away from emotional involvement. It is only when we are helpless that we experience closeness with others, for some of us for the first time. From the broken wrist – that prevents us from functioning in the way we are used to, preparing and making food, driving the car, dressing ourselves – to the patient who is bedridden, the situation creates a need for others to come closer to us. It may be putting an arm around us to guide us to the bathroom, or giving us a bath. In accepting this we also experience our own helplessness, and learn that mere attention from another human being can be a healing experience. We may even learn the pleasure of *not* being in control.

- Being ill can also allow us to express resentments that we have kept secret in the past. We may be able to find angry words for the first time in our lives.

- We may be able to use the time to get in touch with our own body, which we may have ignored since childhood. We can also learn to care for it and nurture it back to health.

- Illness may bring an unsatisfactory way of life to a halt: many 'strong' women find it easier to struggle along in unsatisfactory marriages, looking after house and children with a man who shows them no affection. They find it impossible to ask for help; they believe they do so out of loyalty. In fact, their situation has created a feeling of being always at fault, always unlovable. Or, to take another example, the strong men who keep going in a lifestyle which is obviously depleting their energy, forcing them to feel less and less able, until they collapse into confusion and depression. These men and women might learn, through physical or mental collapse, about what is lacking in their lives, and have time to reassess.

- We can contact – perhaps with the help of a friend, counsellor or therapist – emotions which may surface through day-dreaming. We may be able to experience new aspects of our psyche, to learn to laugh and cry for ourselves.

- We may well, at times like these, be able to recognise our own fears and feelings about death and how these affect our lives. If we can acknowledge these fears it can become a very healing process.
- We can, if we wish, withdraw into an isolation which we may realise is something that we need. The situation makes it possible for us to stay with our own thoughts and needs.
- We may also be able to get in touch with forces within ourselves which we did not know were there. And in so doing we can begin to understand our spiritual and creative nature. This discovery may be the first step towards being able to take part in our own recovery.

It is worth remembering that some illnesses, however hard we try to discover their 'meaning', remain wholly or partly incomprehensible and may well stay with us as chronic states. Perhaps the arthritis I feel in my knee indicates a tension within me which I cannot express without experiencing a tiresome amount of pain and distress? Yet what is it that makes the pain persist, even when I think that I have gained a considerable amount of insight into the matter? It seems that intellectual insight is not enough. And although I can experience relief, sometimes for several days with the help of different forms of alternative healing, the pain always returns. Maybe what is needed is some drastic change in the way I see myself. Though I believe I would go through anything, *anything* to get rid of this damaging and exhausting pain, this clogging of my body which does not allow me to enjoy walking, the condition persists: a stubborn part of my unconscious self will not allow real confrontation.

Attitudes to illness are changing radically. Many doctors are now beginning to view the patient as a whole person, and not just a group of physical ailments. More and more patients may, in the future, be treated in a holistic way: a way which involves the mind, spirit, emotions and body, so that the whole personality will be taken account of during the diagnosis. In terms of this new approach, patients can be involved in their own recovery. We are also beginning to learn and acknowledge the power of the mind and the psyche over the body.

My own experience of working with people who are ill or stressed in other ways makes me believe that reversal of illness, or deep depression, is indeed often possible – without surgical or chemical intervention. Although those who change do need a great deal of loving support, the first step and the most important element is the patient's own desire to take part in that change.

Here we face a difficult question. Does this mean that we are asking those who are ill to take themselves on as patients? Are they expected not only to deal with an exhausting illness, but also to take responsibility for it to the extent that they are expected to 'cure' themselves? That may sound very heartless; in reality it is not quite like that. The first priority, as has been said before, is to recognise our own ability to help ourselves. Without that belief, the way would be hard and frustrating. The more we believe in and acknowledge our own healing powers, the more our bodies will listen and affirm. It is important to see that we need support for this work on ourselves. Often another person's presence is necessary to allow us to see clearly what is happening.

The following are four practical ways a patient can take in seeking to reverse an illness.

1 Find someone to listen

Being listened to is a way of allowing ourselves to look deeply into our own needs. It offers insights by allowing us to examine what has been happening to us in the near and more distant past. It can allow us to make decisions which affect our present lives.

Deep listening is not always possible with close friends and relatives. Too often, they are emotionally involved, especially if the illness is a serious one. This can prevent us from expressing hurts hidden in childhood and carried along for the rest of our lives. If we have not allowed ourselves to grieve properly, or to become angry, or to recognise feelings of rejection, expressing them can be a healing experience.

It is important to find the right person to talk to. Often our intuition, strengthened by being ill, can tell us who that is. Some people have a healing ambiance about them. They could be doctors, psychotherapists, counsellors, or a voluntary counselling service. There are also very useful therapy groups which offer a guided approach to personal problems. Working in a group has the special advantage of allowing us to hear our own problems expressed by others, which can reduce our feelings of isolation.

One very important aspect of being ill is that we are allowed time to be interested in ourselves. Actually, if we think about it, there is nothing more interesting than that, especially if we have spent a lifetime avoiding looking very closely at ourselves. Being listened to, group work, one-to-one counselling offer the support with which to take that on.

2 Relaxation

Working towards recovery involves some kind of relaxation or meditation. These learned techniques help us to contact our unconscious selves and develop strengths affecting our minds and bodies.

The case of Kate is a good illustration of how such relaxation can work. When I first saw her she was clearly under stress. It was Friday and she was due to go into hospital on Wednesday, where a biopsy would be performed on a lump under her arm on Thursday. She talked about her past (she was

40), and explained that she had always feared cancer since her mother had died from breast cancer when she was 18. She examined herself regularly, fearing to find lumps in her own breast. The frightening thing had happened. And it could not have occurred at a worse time. During the last six months her relationship with her husband had so deteriorated that they had decided to divorce. One of her sons was ill and she was worried about the long-term diagnosis. She agreed to learn a form of deep relaxation which took her into a state of 'alpha'. 'Alpha' waves are slow brain waves, which deepen during the practice of relaxation or meditation, but are usually not present in sleep. They produce a state of relaxed awareness. She responded well, and repeated the practice several times before the Wednesday appointment. I saw her on the day she went into hospital. She was cheerful, although understandably still strained. We built into the relaxation an expectation that all would go well, and that she would have a good sleep that night. All very simple. On the Friday I had a letter from her telling me what happened. She slept well without any sleeping tablets and woke feeling refreshed. When the consultant came to examine the place where he was to take the biopsy, the lump had disappeared. He expressed surprise and examined her more closely. Finally, he said: 'There doesn't seem to be anything there. You had better get dressed and go home. Come to see me next week.' She did. Still no sign of the lump. Two years later Kate is happy and well. I saw her for some time after the hospital incident, and clearly she soon needed no more help from me. She had started looking after herself, putting herself first, in fact, for the first time in her life. She changed her diet and took up some of the active sports she had been involved in before she married. Her son recovered quickly with no ill effects. I passed her in the street the other day and hardly recognised her.

There are several ways to reach deep relaxation, from yoga to prayer. It works on two levels. In the body excessive tension can be dangerous. The causes may be many, money worries, relationships, feelings of anxiety or anger. Tension stiffens our muscles, makes for painful joints, as in arthritis, and releases fatty acids into the blood stream. This lowers the immune system, which can allow cancer to invade the body and makes the heart work harder, causing associated problems in the body.

On a deeper level, as we have already mentioned, relaxation and meditative techniques work on our unconscious, gradually making changes in the psyche and affecting the whole of our functioning. It is therefore very important for us to use these techniques to help in our recovery.

3 Healing

In the past, what we know of healing has been associated with the laying on of hands; spiritual healing, or indeed spirit healing. This is not the only way healing can come about. The essential basis of healing is the channelling of energy through the healer to the healed. When being healed, the patient usually feels a change in temperature, a sense of heat or cold, or, sometimes, a faint prickling sensation. Mentally, a state of peace is experienced. At other times there seems to be nothing. Or in other cases a feeling of transcendence may occur.

There is only one energy source for real healers and that is the Mind, the Self, God, Tao; it is called many names. When the energy is moving it moves in waves, and healers are usually in a state of 'alpha'. When an individual has built up patterns in his life not in tune with natural laws he or she becomes ill. At this time healing can be very effective. Healing is not an active therapy; it restores the soul to harmony with cosmic laws. For healing to be effective, there must first be a desire on the part of the patient to accept change. The healer will then be able to unite in empathy with the person being healed. The healer does not heal, but is actually a channel through which energy passes.

Healing, because it restores harmonious energy, is very important. Instantaneous recovery is rare, although it does happen. What is usual is that the patient gains a feeling of peace and hopefulness. Often, a deep refreshing sleep follows a healing session. Healing is also particularly valuable for dying patients. It enables them to approach the end with less discomfort and often without pain. Those who have been able to experience healing at this time seem to contact an inner strength and serenity.

4 Nutrition

The body has material needs and limitations, and for many the experience of illness brings full realisation of the importance of this fact. Many who become ill have not previously taken very real care of themselves, and may well be suffering from poor nutrition as well as its emotional and psychological counterpart. A revision of our attitudes to physical nourishment is not to be underestimated in a culture such as our own. The NACNE (National Advisory Committee on Nutritional Education) Report has shown us that in spite of the wealth of the UK, we are the worst-nourished country in Europe. We eat foods which, far from feeding us, may well be slowly poisoning us.

Until we can fully come to terms with our human limitations, and this must include proper respect for our physical needs – proper nourishment, sleep, relaxation – our innate potential for self-healing will not be accessible to us.

It is in these four areas that we can find ways of meeting illness, even if it appears to be terminal. If there is any meaning in a breakdown in health, hopefully it can encourage suitably radical change. When such change occurs it can enable us as human beings to reach a fuller potential which can bring unexpected richness into our lives, enabling us to appreciate each other and ourselves as never before. It is especially those who have experienced, maybe for the first time, the special charge of love during illness, who talk of being grateful.

Perhaps, even, if we accept that illness allows us to get in touch with our real selves, we might begin to wonder if this is the *only* way. Do we *have* to make such a wearying and painful journey through illness to re-experience what we knew instinctively at birth? Is it, in fact, the best kind of learning situation? Perhaps, if we could begin to live more openly, we could allow ourselves to learn from life in a more sensitive way and we might not always need to reach the impasse that ill-health brings, before being prepared to question our ways.

9 · 'No, I can't do that, my consultant wouldn't like it' ...

JO SPENCE

Jo Spence is an educational photographer and writer whose work has been presented by the BBC's *Arena* and *Omnibus* programmes. She has written for many cultural and photographic journals, as well as co-editing several books on photography. She is currently involved in writing and presenting a series about amateur photography for Channel 4.

Jo Spence's contribution provides an example of her courageous attempt to link ideas and personal experience. As with much of her photographic work, this chapter is autobiographical.

I

In writing about illness it would be easiest for me to take a totally theoretical approach, distancing myself from the reality of its experience, and sheltering instead in the safety of concepts and abstractions – a strategy in which I have frequently sought refuge when dealing with difficult aspects of my professional life as a photographer. But in order to acknowledge my own intimate involvement with illness I feel that I should write in a fully autobiographical and personal mode, so that I can acknowledge what is now happening in my own life as a cancer patient.

Because illness is never simple and seems inextricably bound up with the wider tapestry of my life, I want to attempt to place myself within my family history, and to place that within

a historical and social context. I hope that writing autobiographically will be seen as an invitation to others to try to tease
out their own medical and family histories and not leave it to
professionals to do all the storytelling. Only in this way can
we sow the seeds for learning something new about our
illnesses, ourselves and our potential for change.

I must emphasise before I begin my story that the whole of
my life seems to have been premised on the principle of
conflict. Both within my family and my wider social context it
felt as if there were a continual war going on just beneath the
surface, threatening to break out if certain rituals were not
observed. I needed constantly (though in a way I think this
was quite justifiable) to argue and rebel against what appeared
to be expected of me, to try to be more 'in control'; not only
within the family and at school, but also later at work and in
my partnerships with the opposite sex. When I was silenced, as
I was on many occasions, I learnt other strategies for survival
through 'disobedience': withdrawing my love, withdrawing
my labour, withdrawing my body. I also learnt that I could
wield a form of negative power as an individual, through
illness. In the process, however, I also became alienated from
that centrally evolving core of selfhood, which has only
recently shown itself to be recoverable, in therapy and within
the safety of a new and differently defined loving relationship
formed since I became disabled with cancer.

I did not come to realise until quite recently that life is
inevitably fraught with social and political contradictions and
although it is clearly important that we form alliances and take
political action against social and economic wrongs, we must
not allow these activities to totally undermine our personal
needs. It seems to me absolutely essential that in spite of all the
contradictions of our social existence, we must also nurture an
inner harmony. As I write this I suddenly recall the phrase
spoken some years ago by a wise philosopher of 'keeping your
heart on fire and your head on ice': a combination of feeling
and thinking which many of us find hard to envisage, let alone
practise.

If I allow myself to freely associate around the theme of personal illness, a range of images flows past my mind's eye. Initially all are negative: images of pain, fear, silence, suffering, deprivation, unhappiness and loss through death – memories mostly of people I love, whom I remember as 'victims'. When I try to take these associations deeper, what I 'see' most persistently is my mother – for nobody else has had such an impact on my attitudes to and experience of illness.

Yet as I muse on her presence here, I realise that these impressions are not fixed. In particular, my childhood and adolescent memories of her intermingle with later ones, when I was in hospital with the same illness as her, faced with the possibility of my own imminent death. I remember, for instance, that whenever I visited her in hospital during the final stages of her illness she always seemed very bright and cheerful. Yet I also remember, from my own experience as a patient, that in a ward full of working-class women similar to my mother, many laughed and joked their way through various types of cancer, minimising their own needs – especially when their visitors arrived – afterwards falling back on to their pillows exhausted. In this way friends and families were spared the truth of one another's experience. As the daughter of a suffering woman I learnt to live without compassion and to allow myself to remain in partial ignorance. As I recast my memories of her, I remember the fear in her eyes that she had totally lost control of her life – a fear which I too experienced when I was diagnosed as having breast cancer.

I remember also my guilt, as a daughter, because I could find no way to help her through her various illnesses without giving up what seemed essential to me. My ability to help her seemed inevitably to constellate around taking on some of her chores as a wife and mother. Yet, as my childhood and adolescence had taught me that I could not accept the terms of wife and mother, it is hardly surprising that I found it difficult to be of much use to her at all. I could, perhaps, have offered her love, but my love for her had been in cold storage for so long that I had almost completely lost touch with it.

When I grew up and left the shelter of my parents' home, I remember how I distanced myself from my mother. And just as she did not seem to want to hear about my body, now inextricably bound up with my blossoming sexuality, so she stopped telling me about hers, inevitably threatened by her slowly escalating illnesses. As we tacitly learned to reciprocate each other's silences, so the barriers between us grew.

I do not remember there being any really 'serious' illnesses in my family whilst I was a child, but since then we have, between us, suffered a whole range of afflictions: bronchitis, arthritis, asthma, slipped discs, hardening of the arteries, pneumonia, haemorrhoids, hay fever, and finally cancer. In addition to this we all also suffered recurrent depressive or anxiety states. For these there was a permanent supply of little white pills (later, capsules) in the medicine cupboard. Sometimes one of us would get whisked away into hospital where some minor miracle was performed, about which we understood very little; returning to the family and to the same social and economic conditions and constraints which were no doubt implicated in the illnesses.

It seemed to me that the kind of illnesses my family had, differed very little from those of other families I knew. Neither did the treatments. In some families people just seemed naturally to get more and more ill as they got older, and at some point die: equally mysteriously, at some point new babies arrived. No explanation was ever offered for either event. Going to the doctor, visits to the hospital, seeing consultants and being displayed to the gaze and the prodding fingers of medical students, various forms of drugging and surgery, all seemed the norm. If there were any other approaches to illness they were certainly never talked about in my family. My brother and I soon became children of the welfare state, which promised to look after us from the cradle to the grave. In retrospect, I see our health care as a product of collusion between family circumstances, the medical profession, the state, and the pharmaceutical industry.

In the cultural environment in which I was brought up there

was hardly ever a hint of 'illnesses' specially related to women, except to hear muttered phrases about having a problem 'down there', or of having 'it' 'taken away'. My mother's brief excursion into sex instruction consisted of pointing guardedly at her dressing table drawers and muttering about 'things for mopping up blood', which bewildered me for quite a time (but perhaps I do her an injustice). Links between sexuality and illness were never made explicitly – nor was there any awareness of the fact that women's natural healthy states were continually medicalised because of our ability to menstruate, conceive and bear children. It never occurred to me that there might be anything I personally could 'do' about illness, or that I might have some choice about treatment, until I became a cancer patient at the age of 48. The thought that I could begin to take responsibility for myself or try to look after myself was as remote as the idea of winning the pools. But if I am honest and if there had been a way for me to avoid medical orthodoxy, I know that I would have ignored it, as so much in my life would have needed to be changed – I just would not have known where to start.

I have never really thought more than superficially about my body until fairly recently, except to be ashamed of the way I looked, allowing myself only a kind of passive sexuality in darkened bedrooms with the men I have loved. I was totally ignorant about the way in which my body functioned, its material needs, its symbiotic relationship to the world, and the need for harmony in my life. I just knew that I had to 'look good' and perform in a variety of ways, as a woman, in order to be loved. For all the strengths of growing up in a working-class family, living in a north London suburb, it did not prepare me in any way to be able to take on serious research, engage in abstract thinking, or make long term plans for anything. Such things had to wait until I had become middle class, and learnt those ways within higher education.

Within family life my brother and I seemed to be expected to respond constructively to whatever life brought us, rather than being able to take any action on our own account or define our individual sexuality and living patterns differently from our parents. This was a continuing cause of conflict for us all, and was clearly implicated in 'nervous' illnesses and stress patterns right across the family (phenomena which would no doubt be considered relevant in current family therapy). As the family group became more and more diseased I just awaited my turn to inevitably become ill.

My parents were very politicised about economics and the struggle between labour and capital. My father was a Branch Secretary in his trade union, and spent numerous hours of his time fighting for people's rights at work, and especially for sickness benefits and payments for industrial injuries. Yet he always put his union work before his own health, never, apparently, having any inkling of how he could have helped us as a family to have 'better' or healthier lives. My mother, for her part, did the 'double shift' as factory worker and housewife for thirty or so years. She filled us lovingly with old-fashioned, fatty stodge – which we all loved – and inculcated in me obsessive habits of domestic and personal hygiene.

In my family, perhaps only because of the class position into which we were born, there was very little concept of 'free choice'. Both of my parents had to take whatever jobs were on offer from the nearby industrial estate: they did not plan 'careers' for themselves, though they did attempt to do so for my brother and myself. We lived where cheap housing was available, attended the statutory local state school and used the nearest 'panel' doctor.

Both of my parents grew up in a world where jobs were never plentiful, and people seemed to prosper only under the influence of the old-fashioned work ethic. It seems to me now that both of them literally worked themselves to death. Because they were so hard-up (though they never openly acknowledged themselves to be 'poor') they both continued working long after the official retirement age. Now, as I write, I remember my father coming in from his tiring job as a storekeeper in a local engineering company, still working in his late sixties, lungs exploding with the phlegm of chronic bronchitis, gasping for breath, lips blue, nose and cheeks glowing with the ruddiness of tiny broken veins – and proud that he had walked the distance of three bus stops in order to save tuppence from the family budget. At the time I did not value what he did. He never told hard luck stories or saw himself as a victim, but was always the hero of the underdog. Yet, even though both of my parents fought all their lives against the system they found themselves caught up in – through the Labour Party and their respective trade unions – they had very little consciousness of the politics of family life, with its uneven and repressive power relationships.

Illness in my family usually meant a complete breakdown of social relations. Both of my parents worked full-time in industry, leaving for work at 6 a.m. and returning twelve hours later. Everything had to be organised around that. For my parents, being 'off sick' meant a drastic drop in income (something I did not really understand and constantly moaned about when I was a child), whilst for me it meant the forgoing of certain rights and privileges. My brother and I were both latch-key children for a large part of our early years, though the impact of this was different for each of us. For me it often meant doing jobs that my mother had no time to do; small things in addition to everyday helping, like running errands, ironing, making beds, tidying up, washing up, doing the vegetables for the evening meal. Though this does not sound impressive, it took up an enormous amount of my precious time. For my brother, on the other hand, this entailed very little loss of freedom; there was always his older sister to be the buffer, clear up the mess and be responsible.

I played the role of a surrogate parent with no reciprocal benefits. This experience laid the groundwork for always putting the needs of others before my own – something which I have had to come to terms with in later life. When my mother finally admitted to us that she was ill, there were further duties; in addition to running for the doctor and collecting prescriptions from the chemist it meant having to stay in more often, with additional anxiety of her being at home whilst I attempted to do jobs 'badly'. Many is the time she crossed the landing from the bedroom to the bathroom, wheezing and coughing and yet remarking on her way that the hall was rather dusty, or that I had not polished the brass very well!

The rooms in their small flat were all in close proximity to one another and there was very little privacy anywhere. The bathroom door was never left unlocked when in occupation and, except when we were small children, my parents' bedroom was strictly off limits. I shared a bedroom with my brother until I left home. When I reached puberty, token privacy was conceded necessary by the addition of a small room divider which my father built into our bedroom. Bodies were never celebrated in our family, and as we became more self-conscious as adolescents, we went through nightly charades of undressing secretly and 'not looking' at each other. I have no recollections either of ever seeing my father's or my mother's body, except on the occasion when my mother, lying supine in her hospital bed, called us around her to see her scar. (With hindsight, I now see that we were invited to inspect what she now lacked – her breast.)

Although illness did not in actual fact occupy a vast amount of family time when we were children, I now see that in memory it has taken on gigantic proportions, forming the central story to which all other experiences relate. For me it became an important part of the matrix of ways in which I express myself. Initially I suffered from asthmatic attacks, which offered relief from stressful situations, conflict, and environmental factors beyond my control. It also served to win attention from parents who were often absent when needed, because of the demands of working life. A little later I suffered from psychosomatic or allergic states such as wheezing, sneezing, skin eruptions and anxiety states; for all these seemed to be accepted as 'okay' illnesses in my family. On the other hand, the illnesses of my parents were for me, as a child, often just a damned nuisance, and I had no idea of the hardship and anxiety they went through in order to maintain normal appearances for as long as possible during such periods.

When we were older these patterns of disease began to strangle the family, locking us into negative relationships whose tangled knots seemed impossible to unravel. Given the fact that habit is so insidious – witness the effort to give up even the tiniest addiction – it is not surprising that it took a cataclysmic event like cancer to bring me to my senses and to try to begin to re-assemble my sense of self.

WAR TIME

In my family there was no mythology of the good times of war. My father was too old to be called up and anyway would have been exempted as he suffered from persistent haemorrhoids (though they never caused a day's absence from industrial work). Family life shattered after war broke out in 1939. I was evacuated three times, constantly moved schools and changed homes eight times. My parents moved jobs, having to be separated from the rest of the family, and my brother and I were 'minded' during holidays. All of this is of course on top of the actual trauma of armed conflict, air raids, fear of attack and enemy occupation, food shortages and rationing. There was some compensation for me, for I was able to roam, free from parental control, and learned to survive both alone and in groups. The fact that this survival often took the form of stealing and lying was never a cause for celebration. But though it was not seen as legitimate revolt, our inadequacy of means did nevertheless provide a certain justification.

We were none of us expected to express our anxiety or grief about these upheavals or separations. In retrospect, I do not therefore find it surprising that within a year of the war ending I was sent to the local hospital because of prolonged bouts of asthma. Although psychosomatic causes were suggested (for example that I had repressed my fears during wartime) the white-coated specialist seemed benevolent enough as he suggested various ways in which we could deal chemically with asthma 'attacks'. Later I was one of the early guinea pigs for steroid treatment and consequently developed a 14 lb ovarian tumour and was out of action for nearly three months. I nevertheless still supposed that everybody had done their best for me. When spots 'broke out' all over my body, various ointments were experimented with. And when we 'did battle' to quell the hayfever, it is hardly surprising that I still did not think to question the medical profession's continuing use of war rhetoric to describe my condition. It seemed to me already that the body was a battlefield (dare I say, the enemy) and that the medical profession provided the ammunition with which to win through. In retrospect I find this an alarming inheritance.

GROWING UP IS GROWING INTO

In the early 1970s both my mother, then my father, died quite suddenly. I felt great sadness – and relief – that the masquerade of being a 'good daughter' was over (with all the sexual repression that it had entailed). It was not until I was ill in hospital with breast cancer that I began to remember how I had helped the family doctor with my own mother's euthanasia whilst she was suffering from liver cancer some six weeks after the removal of her breast. I was the one who was, again, sent to the chemist – this time to collect a bottle of colourless fluid which we were to administer to her orally once she had begun to go into a coma which the doctor had induced by injection. There had been no family counselling, nor discussion with her or my aged father, who was so shattered by her death that he died within three weeks, of heart failure. The decision had been made – it seemed like lightning – and acted upon equally quickly. Although I was grateful at the time that such a humane doctor had looked after us for so many years, it is very difficult to come to terms with now. I had in many ways completely disavowed her death, never questioning it. Now I not only have to come to terms with hers, but also with the possibility of my own.

After my parents died I used their tiny inheritance to buy myself the luxury of some time in which I did not have to work. I took a year off and felt for the first time in my life the difference between having to work continuously to support myself, often when I didn't want to or felt too ill, and being able to make decisions knowing that, for a short while at least, I could survive financially without going under. I resolved never to get into the situation my parents had always been in; poor, stressed, caught up in an ethos of 'respectability', and with a daughter who wanted to opt out of family life for as far back as she could remember. My brother, for his part, moved to Devon and endeavoured to live his fantasy of the rural dream with his wife and two children until he could no longer get a job because of the economic depression. His splendid health, a matter for some pride in our family, gradually broke down as his life fell to pieces through divorce, loss of children, loss of home, low income and long working hours in temporary factory work. Slowly his lungs began to give out with asthma and bronchitis...and he eventually succumbed to depression. All this was treated expediently and chemically without any form of counselling. He will now be on drugs for the rest of his foreseeable life.

In my thirties, I became ambitious. By now I was a high street portrait photographer instead of a secretary and worked purely for the satisfaction and pleasure in what I and others could learn through it, rather than having to treat it purely economically. I began to be involved with the children's rights movement and worked towards a group practice within photography. I began to experience the first glimmerings of how I might overcome my 'inferiority complex' about my lack of education. I began to concentrate on finding out more about the subject in which I was so profoundly interested – photography. I attended conferences, workshops, joined reading groups, learned to give lectures, ran evening classes, became co-editor of a magazine, helped with others to set up a charity for photographic education, co-published a book, set up endless projects, became a writer, and so on. Over a period of fifteen years I became a completely obsessive workaholic caught up in various campaigns and struggles. Eventually, because of ethical qualms about earning a living through

documenting the misery of others, I decided to apply to the
Polytechnic of Central London to become a mature student on
a degree course which dealt with the theory and practice of
photography. After a three-year struggle to learn, I emerged
with my first class Honours degree. My parents would have
been proud of me. Two months after leaving college I was
diagnosed as having breast cancer.

II

For as long as I can remember I have negotiated change: jobs,
homes, lovers (and especially my mind!). Since childhood I
have lived with a 'conflict' model of life, a model in which
battle and war were natural, and an essential means to survival.
The 'ammunition' for such warfare in my own life was never
physical violence though, but rather a coercion in the form
of words; the silencing of my needs, through innuendo, fear of
the withdrawal of love, or threats of punishment. My
strategies in situations of extreme adversity were very limited –
either to disavow what was happening to me, and walk away;
or to confront everything head-on, and rebel against it in a
very self-destructive way. I suppose, in some respects too, I
was my parents' daughter, in that coming from a socialist
household I often spoke out against the adversity of others –
whilst at the same time ignoring my own! However, I never
felt safe enough either to abandon or to challenge my parents
in any concrete way, until I reached the age of 25. I then,
suddenly decided to leave home – causing a major upheaval
within family life from which, in some ways, none of us ever
recovered. This pattern extended to all later relationships: I
would try for a while to negotiate my needs and if they could
not be met then I just left, or became silent.

The one exception to this pattern was my ever-present
relationship with the medical profession to whom I had,
unthinkingly, allocated god-like status and a mantle of
infallibility. I was naive and trusting for a long time, colluding
in the unequal power relationship which any systematised

witholding of knowledge brings about. I hung on to my infantalisation, like a crutch, in spite of my health steadily worsening over the years. Asthmatics must be very 'low reward' patients for the medical profession. In my case there was never any prolonged respite, just bouts of asthma and related illnesses, escalating across the years, as did the intake of chemical treatments and consequent side-effects. I see now that I always went to doctors and consultants with my hand held out, waiting for another 'fix' to carry me through until the next visit. The contradiction – between this dependence and yet at the same time feeling that I had such apparent independence within social and emotional relationships – never really became obvious until I was in therapy. Here I was able to examine the split between my mind and my body: my generalised feelings of powerlessness; the fears which lay behind my obsession to be 'in control' of my mind – whilst clearly at the same time out of control of my health. Above all, I began to question my unexpressed anger towards the world, and in particular to the medical profession, at not having anything positive to offer me as a breast-cancer patient.

It was not until I began to research into the politics of cancer that the pharmaceutical industry finally came into focus. I began to make connections between the apparent financial saving to the state giving drugs in order to get people 'back on their feet' and economically viable again as quickly as possible, as opposed to the long-term, and perhaps less profitable idea of finding more radical and organic alternatives to 'magic bullets'. I began to search for other types of health care. I began to reflect, too, upon the fact that, given the incidence of suicide, depression, drug dependence, cigarette and alcohol addiction, as well as family breakdown, among the medical profession it is extraordinary that they appear to not want to open up any sort of dialogue with patients about the potential for sharing of power and responsibility for health (with implications, of course, for their own). The fact that, as a culture, we are socialised to be dependent upon doctors and on drugs for maintaining our health and ultimate survival, rather than examining ways of making our lives and the environment a healthier place to live in is, surely, a nightmare we have all somehow blundered into?

PROFESSIONAL HEAL THYSELF

To shift now into my own field – photography – I believe that the relationships I had with clients and the artefacts I made were expressions of ways in which I tried to speak to people. Originally, as a high street photographer, I offered my 'gifts' to members of the public who paid me in order to provide them with images of idealised family life which would support the idea that all families are 'happy' and that thus my clients were 'good parents'. Later, as a documentary photographer, I began to teach and petition for social change. I then turned my hand to 'agitprop' photography: to propagandise and ask political questions. When I became a mature student, my photographs and theoretical work were a means to academic viability and professional power. In contrast to this, when I became ill in 1982, I began to use photography for myself instead of other people, and it became a way of having a dialogue with myself, or re-visioning illness, and asking new questions. (Later, when I developed with others the idea of photo-therapy I was quite happy to make such work publicly available; but initially it was just for myself.)

I had always assumed that I would be different from my parents; yet I soon began to realise, through the expression of this interior dialogue in pictures, that I had followed in their footsteps, and had, after all, failed to look after myself. Although I had, unlike them, in some senses acquired personal power through my profession, my workaholism, with its emphasis on developing my intellect – though it took a different form from theirs, which has been based on economic survival – was nevertheless a similar pattern. The attendant and total neglect of my bodily needs had resulted in a slow, grinding breakdown, like a weary old horse plodding under a massive workload. In my capacity as a photo-therapist I have begun to develop a professional practice in which it is possible now to have a dialogue with my clients; in which they use my skills in order to learn more about themselves and their social/cultural environment so that they can become able to make more informed choices about their lives. This is in distinct contrast to my other photographic practices which were about maintaining the status quo, or trying to persuade others to change the world.

By using photography, throughout my illness, it has meant that certain facets of my history were planted squarely and visibly in front of me. Facing up, at last, to the knowledge that my mother had died six weeks after the removal of a breast, at least in part due to her liver cancer not being diagnosed, my faith in orthodox medicine vanished. I now found myself in conflict with the medical profession. I finally found the courage to say that I wanted minimal surgery, no chemotherapy or irradiation (even though I was told that I was virtually signing my own death warrant). I suddenly found myself having said 'No', yet with nowhere else to go. I knew nothing!

Thus began a journey of self-discovery – as it has been for many others – starting at the Bristol Cancer Help Centre. From it has come a complete restructuring, permeating every part of my life. I have rejected a medical profession whose basic metaphors of disease are those of WAR: to cut, burn and chemically destroy the 'problem'; to get rid of the 'trouble' (in my case a malignant tumour); to knife it out whilst not encouraging me to ask why it is there. These practices seemed to me to be similar to the ways in which the state tends to intervene in other 'trouble spots': social unrest or rioting, for example, when one must get rid of the 'problem', drive it underground, and hope that it will go away.

How can the function of illness be investigated in our individual lives? Given that research has indicated, for example, that 90 per cent of known cancers are preventable, and if such cancer is the embodiment of psychic, social and environmental dis-eases then it makes little sense for the medical profession to merely remove or obliterate such 'signs and symptoms' when our bodies 'speak out'. And if patients, as a result of treatment *only* of their symptoms – ignoring their feelings of helplessness and their fear – become psychologically disturbed or depressed, and yet they receive only *further* psychotropic chemical drugging, is it hardly surprising that they do not find it easy to begin to define and articulate new needs, for which they need a voice, either individually or collectively.

SOME LESSONS TO BE LEARNED

If I were to ask myself the one thing that I have learned as a result of having cancer it is just simply that I never realised how powerless I really was, and how few rights in the world I had, until a young man in a white coat, whom I had never seen before, surrounded by others similarly clad, stopped at my bedside in a provincial English hospital, ruffled through some notes clamped to a board, leaned over me and drew a large black cross above my breast, uttering those memorable words: 'That's the one that is coming off!' From that moment on I was on total alert. I began to search for a treatment which would recognise me as a whole human being, and not as parts to be disposed of; one that would take account of my physical, psychic, social and spiritual self. I even investigated my legal position in relation to suicide and euthanasia.

In the end I opted for a practice in north London which offered me traditional Chinese Medicine, linked to Jungian therapy. Strange bedfellows! These two practitioners have gradually induced in me the desire to better love myself and to take proper account of my needs. From this starting point I could begin again to relate with others. Traditional Chinese Medicine is an integrated system of treatment in which diet, exercise, acupuncture, massage, forms of meditation and weekly herbal decoctions are offered. This treatment is available as *one* of the choices for breast-cancer patients in China and has a long history. It is not available on the National Health Service nor is it being systematically investigated by any of the major hospitals. It does not offer a 'cure', but I am pleased with the way in which it has fitted into my life and allowed me a relatively normal life in the last few years.

Right from the start of this particular illness I realised that there was to be no magical cure for the ways in which I had unknowingly abused my body with bad diet, lack of rest, overstress, over-work, continual conflict and unhappiness. In that sense then, I was not seeking a cure, but merely a way of learning to live differently and more harmoniously, within myself and with others. But how is it possible to transform my conflict model of life, when I see massive injustices and inequalities – in relation to people's race, gender, sexuality, class, age and abilities – systematically and institutionally maintained?

How could I begin to go about unravelling this problem? My first change was in my diet: out went all the junk food which I loved so much, and in came a 'clean' semi-vegan diet. I gave up battling to hold together an eleven-year relationship which provided neither of us with any peace and very little love, although my partner was very supportive in every way he knew. Through long sessions with counsellors I began to discharge my anger and grief (mostly for myself in the early stages). I began to do some research, so that I should no longer be merely saying 'no', but would be informed of the alternatives. This knowledge I eventually shared, by writing articles in magazines and through making a travelling exhibition of other approaches to breast cancer (see references). I found this entire subject to be a minefield of taboos and ignorance. Each year in the UK 15,000 women die of the advanced stages of cancer, stemming initially from breast cancer for which there are hardly any counselling resources available – needed more than ever now that it is being recognised by the patients that there are controversial and conflicting attitudes among consultants about treatment. The major charity to help breast cancer sufferers is called the Mastectomy Association as though the two – breast cancer and mastectomy – were synonymous.

I began also to question how I used my energy, and remembered graphically the wise words of an old friend who had said to me 'at least peace, at most joy'. I had seen this as an enigma; the significance of the words escaped me, but I now began to reflect on them differently. In talking to a psycho-therapist about the way in which I saw my body as 'the enemy' and 'having let me down', she gently pointed out that my body was my best friend and had stood with me through thick and thin, in spite of my obvious inability to listen to her often repeated signs and symptoms as a way of communicating with me.

At this point in time my breast had again become dis-eased, and clearly cancer had come back on to the site of the scar. Instead of disavowing that I was ill, I began to take my breast literally into my own hands, to cradle her and to talk to her. David, my new partner in life, responded similarly. We began in our physical life together to mutually exchange whole body massage, gently easing away years of tension, trying to open ourselves out, to communicate in different ways. We set up a pattern of counselling each other, so that we could try to deal with ongoing anxiety, problems and grief, though this is not always easy. We found new patterns for using our time beneficially and joyfully together, rather than always working and then collapsing at weekends. He began to share the same diet as myself and eventually we ceased to think of it as a diet but more as a way of life. Although initially I had experienced a physical and emotional breakdown, when the time came to reconstruct my life in a way which could reap the benefits of hard research work, I had only to negotiate with my partner's needs, for we had no children to consider. In this respect perhaps it was an easier task than for some people with children or families to look after, as we were able to re-invent our own lives within the limitations only of our income and social expectations.

Because we had both decided to continue intermittently with therapy of one sort or another (we met at a therapeutic weekend) we have been able to investigate much of our past lives, our patterns of neurotic behaviour, ways in which our sexuality had been defined for us, and ways in which we had inherited both the eating and stress patterns of our separate families.

Though money undeniably sets limits to the type of health care you can purchase for yourself outside the National Health Service, we have not, in fact, spent a lot of money on therapy. We learnt to co-counsel in a local evening class and then joined the network of counsellors who work freely together. This has been supplemented by some well-chosen paid sessions with therapists specialising in working with cancer patients, or those with health problems. As a result of all this we now feel we have more choices; that we are not merely responding, but can actively participate in shaping our own lives. Although I am not 'better', my regime continues, my work as a photographer is flourishing, and we are already planning how to survive on a low income if redundancy or retirement comes. It is not an easy life, but it is one in which we feel less vulnerable and less powerless.

SOME TENTATIVE CONCLUSIONS

Illness is usually spoken about in terms of victims and heroes, especially in relation to cancer. If you are terminally ill you are a victim, but if you managed 'against all odds' to survive both the treatment and the disease, then you are a hero or heroine. This drama can be seen daily in the media and is merely *one* way of understanding the meanings of this particular illness. It is, in fact, a very limiting way of defining illness. Thinking back to my own family history, it was not like that: illnesses participated as a theme in the long, hard struggle with the structures which defined the patterns of our lives and relationships. For me, within my own illnesses, learning to 'just be' instead of continually responding and reacting to outside stimulus has been the most difficult path for me to follow. Letting go of responsibility for the needs of others was perhaps one of my most difficult challenges. This does not of course negate the continual need for the struggle for better health care in an organised, political way. Most people are not as privileged as I am.

Because this is not a story with a 'happy ending', I can only say that I now live my life from day to day but with a long-term sense of looking after myself and others in more aware ways. Because I have learned so much since I became ill I am both more sceptical about how it is possible to bring about major changes in our lives, and more hopeful because of the extraordinary people I have met in the field of holistic health. I do feel though, that there are some grounds for optimism about a more patient-centred attitude to illness and health, both because patients are beginning to demand it, and because there are indications that some elements of the medical profession are also shifting the terms of their involvement.

So, a final question which arises for me is this: given that we live in a culture which is dominated by metaphors of war; given that our bodies, (women's in particular), are so fragmented through advertising, pornography and the fetishisms of fashion; given that we are taught that the mind is separate from the body, and that state schooling and medicine institutionalise a split between thinking and doing, theory and practice; given that we live under such stress in order to survive; given that we have to struggle to define for ourselves our potential to reshape cultural definitions for our sexuality, gender roles, race, class and power relations – how can we begin to orientate ourselves towards acquiring the social understanding and potency which would enable us to lead less conflict-ridden lives? Starting, perhaps with a patient-centred medicine and child-centred education?

How can we begin to move on from the speciality-centred, consultant-dominated, hierarchical, drug- and surgery-based, cost-effective medicine? How do we learn to move beyond keeping quiet and appearing to be grateful for whatever we are offered, pleasing 'our consultant'? People, when actually offered *choices*, cease saying 'No, I can't do that, my consultant wouldn't like it', as I have so often heard. How can we forge a social environment which will encourage us to ask questions and gain the relevant knowledge, so that we can contribute towards taking more responsibility for our own minds and bodies – frightening as that may seem?

I have written autobiographically when I could have written from a purely theoretical point of view, because I believe this is the key to real communication and hence to a social policy in our speech. I believe that it is possible to transform our lives and the relationships we are involved in, given the environment, access to relevant knowledge, and the will to unravel the identities we inhabit – *and* for us to be able to function at our best, *even* if we are dying. If it *is* possible to begin to take some responsibility for making informed decisions about our bodies and our lives – even with such an 'impossible' illness as cancer – then hopefully this will offer itself as a model for other seemingly impossible types of personal, political and social struggle. We cannot continue to live with our eyes, ears and mouths shut.

In my twin capacity, both as a patient and a professional photographer, I can acknowledge and share, as well as the pain and the fear, the extraordinary pleasure and inventiveness of the disease which my fate is bound up with and, paradoxically, the very positive effects it has had on my life. Of course I would have preferred it to have been easier, but that would have been another story!

References

The Picture of Health? Alternative Approaches to Breast Cancer is a widely acclaimed travelling exhibition of photographs and text, put together by Jo Spence with the assistance of Rosy Martin and Maggie Murray. It is available for hire or loan from the Cockpit Gallery, Princeton Street, London WC1.

Putting Myself in the Picture, a personal, political and photographic autobiography, published by Camden Press, 1986.

10 · No answer to Job: reflections on the limitations of meaning in illness

ADOLF GUGGENBÜHL-CRAIG
and
NIEL MICKLEM

Adolf Guggenbühl-Craig is a Swiss psychiatrist. He studied theology and medicine in Zurich and Paris, and trained in psychiatry in the USA and Switzerland. He then became a Jungian analyst and now has a psychiatric and analytical practice in Zurich in partnership with Dr Niel Micklem. Guggenbühl-Craig is a member of the curatorium of the C. G. Jung Institute in Zurich and a lecturer and training analyst. He is the former president of the International Association of Analytical Psychology and he is the author of *Power and the Helping Professions, Marriage Dead or Alive* and *Eros on Crutches* (all by Spring Publications).

Niel Micklem is an English physician educated in medicine in Oxford and London. After some years of practice, he turned to psychotherapy and later studied at the C. G. Jung Institute in Zurich. He is a lecturer and training analyst at the Institute and practices in partnership with Dr Guggenbühl-Craig.

The title 'The Meaning of Illness' suggests that each of us may, and even perhaps should, find 'meaning' in our illnesses. Adolf Guggenbühl-Craig and Niel Micklem warn against a cult of meaning, which may shield its followers from a realisation of the inescapably tragic dimension to illness.

I – Adolf Guggenbühl-Craig

Our ability to enjoy life and to live fully depends very much on a healthy and well-functioning body. When illness enters our lives, the possibility of us functioning according to our abilities, inclinations and desires is greatly hindered.

Illness, like catastrophes and disasters, always arouses our need for an explanation. Ethnographers tell us that in archaic society illness was considered to be the result of bewitchment by either an evil power or an evil person. In many parts of Europe witches were until recently suspected of causing disease. Jews were supposed to have poisoned the water and caused the plague in the Middle Ages. Or could it be that God himself punished and still punishes sinners with diseases as He punished mankind with floods, fires and earthquakes?

This tendency to add insult to injury can be found in the Bible; in the Book of Job, for instance. Job was a God-fearing, pious and moral man. He was struck by bad luck, lost all his possessions, and became seriously ill. The friends who visited him insisted that he must have been a great sinner, and that his misfortunes must be the punishment of God.

We of the twentieth century have certainly moved beyond this moralistic view of sickness. Or have we?

Let us look at medicine, the science of disease. The classical orthodox medicine of the nineteenth and twentieth centuries has tried to understand disease and illness from a purely 'scientific' point of view and thus religion, morals and psychology have been banned from its discipline. The human body has been more or less understood as a very complicated machine, a refined computer with a superb chemical factory. This unbelievably complex mechanism can be disturbed for all kinds of reasons, and the function of medicine is to find out the mechanical, chemical and other causes of the disfunction, and repair it. This approach has shown impressive results.

At the beginning of the twentieth century, psychology began to raise its head. Many doctors were no longer satisfied with the purely mechanical and chemical approach to disease.

They tried to understand and explain physical disease according to the psychological background of the sick person. Psychosomatic medicine began to flourish and behind many diseases certain psychological disturbances were suspected. Some diseases were obviously psychosomatic and experiments with animals and human beings confirmed this. Excessive anger and frustration, for example, change the composition of gastric juices and cause ulcers; too much tension leads to high blood pressure. The connection between some psychological conditions and physical diseases, now closely observed, could not be denied. But, these positive experimental results caused a flood of psychosomatic fantasies. Unexplainable diseases like cancer began to be understood psychologically. Eventually it became possible to 'understand' every disease symbolically and psychologically. For instance arteriosclerosis – the narrowing of the arteries – was connected to having a narrow psychological outlook; cancer of the breast was understood as the result of a 'negative attitude towards femininity' and so forth.

When we look at the explanations given by psychosomatic medical doctors today, we make a strange discovery; every disease seems to be a kind of punishment for a particular sin in the sense of the sick person having an unbalanced psychological development. We seldom hear that someone falls ill because he is psychologically well-balanced, because he is able to express feelings in a fruitful way or because he is a loving and caring person.

The results of the attempt to understand the body, its functions and dysfunctions as a symbolic expression of the life of the psyche, as a language of the soul, are fruitful and stimulating. These are, however, mainly fantasy. Psychosomatic explanations show their fantastic nature by the fact that they are seldom scientifically verified. It is practically impossible to demonstrate statistically that patients with, for instance, coronary diseases are of a specific psychological nature. Most psychosomatic explanations are 'proven' by anecdotes. Psychological typologies of people suffering from various diseases come and go. First, managers were supposed to be prone to high blood pressure, then the assistant managers, frustrated by the fact that they were not managers. Ambition was supposed to be behind each case, but we may then ask why some groups of lumberjacks suffer from high blood pressure. Are they over-ambitious too?

The disturbing feature is not the fantasy aspect of psychosomatic medicine, but its all-pervasive *moralism*. All these beautiful modern symbolic explanations are harmful in their very *moralism*. Sick people, people with cancer for instance, with dreadful infections, with chronic diseases like arteriosclerosis, not only have to suffer, but are made to feel guilty as well: their diseases are entirely their own fault; they have failed to develop psychologically; they have suppressed their feelings or have not suppressed them enough; they have been too friendly or not friendly enough.

This psychosomatic moralism is harmful in more ways than one. Not only does it create sinners, but pharisees as well and the sinners are looked down upon by the pharisees. How often we hear colleagues talk in a condescending way about their patients with so-called psychosomatic diseases.

Before continuing, it is important to avoid misunderstanding by distinguishing clearly between a moral and a *moralistic* attitude. The latter is a perversion or caricature of the former. We can never be moral enough. Morality attempts to follow eros, to obey guide-lines which help us to do more good than evil. Moralism, however, abuses these guide-lines and harms. The pharisee is moralistic and uses moral guide-lines to put everyone else down.

In our approach to disease could we not find more courage to be *agnostic*? We do not know what human life is all about and in particular we do not know what disease is all about. We can stand this lack of knowing as long as life, individually or collectively, runs smoothly. However, when catastrophe hits, in the form of disease and illness, this lack of knowing what life – and disease – are all about becomes unbearable.

It is not too much to say the Book of Job is one of the greatest psychological and religious works of all times. We are told by experts that the beginning and the end of this Book are later additions. The original story, so they claim, tells only how the pious, moral and God-fearing man was struck by disaster and disease. His friends suspected he must be a sinner being punished by God for his sins, but Job rejected the accusations. He simply did not understand why he had to suffer so much, why God had sent him all this misery. When God eventually spoke to him, he gave no explanations. He pointed out simply that he, God, had created everything, rules everything, and that there was no explanation to be given.

The beginning of the story, when God makes a bet with Satan that he will not be able to corrupt his faithful servant Job, is – as mentioned – probably an addition. It dilutes the frightening tale, trying to give it some sense and taking off the hard edges. But the core of the story has to be seen in the 'answer' of God to Job. It is no answer at all. God does not give any explanation for Job's sufferings.

The Book of Job is remarkable because it tries to look at catastrophe, misery, disease and suffering without trying to give any explanation, moralistic or otherwise. It simply relates how God behaved, and gives no explanation.

Disease has to be taken as a tragedy, as a dreadful happening without meaning or purpose. That should perhaps be our first approach. It does not mean, however, that we cannot make something of illness once it appears. An ambitious salesman, for instance, does not catch hepatitis in order to be forced to slow down because his ambitions are psychologically sinful. But once he is ill, having to rest, he may use his time to reflect more. That we can sometimes turn a disease into an advantage does not mean that the disease happened *because* we have sinned psychologically. But, in the spirit of 'making the best of it', disease, taken as a tragedy, as an inexplicable act of God or of nature, could give us something. We Jungian psychologists consider individuation to be as important as well-being or health, and by individuation we mean not only becoming a conscious individual, but experiencing the transcendental aspect of life, getting in touch with the self, with our divine spark as well.

Might not the transcendental aspect of individuation be fostered by facing the apparent meaninglessness of catastrophes, by facing diseases mainly as a tragedy just as Job had to face his misery and sickness as a completely incomprehensible act of God?

By doing this, we might individuate in the sense of getting in touch with the divine spark, just as Job did, when he felt that his misery, his disease, had no meaning and was certainly not the result of his being a sinner. The reward of his attitude was that in the end God at least *spoke* to him, not to explain what it was all about, but to show his existence.

Job after all was fortunate for he talked to God and God to him. What more could any human being wish for? How many of us can claim that God has talked to us personally? If being able to bear the tragic meaninglessness of disease results in hearing God speak, then the dreadful experience was worthwhile.

This may come across as a total rejection of psychosomatic mythology, its beautiful and aesthetic symbolism. It is not so much that such a mythology has no use, but that it has definite limitations.

All psychosomatic theories and fantasies, all psychosomatic mythologies are touching expressions of a deep faith in life. We cannot understand disease, suffering and catastrophes, but we can religiously believe that in the end all the dreadful things we have to experience have a transcendental meaning. So we elaborate beautiful aesthetic explanations for all the misery we experience and thereby express symbolically that we believe all might make sense in the end. Psychosomatic theories have to be understood as legends which hint at the transcendental side of all our suffering, of all our disease. Psychosomatic fantasies are only absurd if they are taken as scientific explanations and not as mythologies.

There is a gnostic and an agnostic way to deal with sickness – or should we say, more simply a 'knowing' and a 'not knowing' way. Both are legitimate and both have their advantages and disadvantages. Today psychosomatic medicine is inclined to be gnostic, to 'know' the meaning of illness, at least the symbolic meaning. So a whole psychosomatic mythology has developed, sometimes based on a few hints given by scientific medicine. It is, however, usually pure poetry. This psychosomatic poetry has a function as intimated earlier, but we must bear in mind that agnostic psychosomatic medicine also has its function and is valuable. Here no legends are told; the inexplicable tragedy of disease is faced squarely after the manner of Job, and hopefully we reach another psychological level of individuation – as Job did, through acknowledging that God gave him no answer, but *spoke* to him.

Gnostic and agnostic psychosomatic medicine can be compared to the two extreme ways in which Christians and disciples of other religions have tried to understand God. Some have prayed in the desert with nothing around them but sand and wasteland; others in churches filled with elaborate and beautiful pictures and statues depicting the glory of God.

It cannot be denied that the body often wants to tell us something, though it is difficult to know what. And is it always a moralistic tale? It seems sometimes as if really unpleasant and very unconscious people enjoy good health until ripe old age, while those who are friendly and especially conscious suffer all kinds of aggravating diseases. Maybe unpleasantness and unconsciousness are healthy.

Has the time not come to get rid of the *moralism in psychosomatic mythology*? One of the simplest and most childish ways to understand what happens to us human beings is to see it in a moralistic frame work. 'The good people are rewarded and the wicked will be punished.' This is the gist of hundreds of cowboy movies and many detective stories. However, even this 'good guy is rewarded and the bad guy punished' mythology is not entirely wrong. It underlines in a touching and naive way the importance of morality. It is so tremendously important to be moral; life without morals would be hell;

where the law of the jungle rules there can be no happiness and no psychological development.

So the moralistic psychosomatic mythologies have their usefulness, however limited. With simple tales they underline the extreme importance of morals.

But do not the disadvantages of the moralistic psychosomatic mythology outweigh the advantages? They reinforce, for instance, in an unfortunate way our cumbersome and fruitless guilt feelings which are at the root of many neuroses. We may hope, therefore, that our colleagues in psychosomatic medicine will continue to develop their tales and legends and find ever more fantastic stories about the background of disease, but will leave moralism out.

How pleasing it will be when, one day, these psychosomatic colleagues tell beautiful stories about the connections of psychologically well-balanced, healthy individuals and when, for instance in cancer, they show how not only psychological sinners but others too can just as well be struck by disaster. Tragedies reflect life as much as uplifting moral tales. The body has to be listened to carefully, but its language varies and its message is seldom simple.

II – Niel Micklem

Gild the farthing where you will, it remains a farthing still. The same may be said to apply to illness in the context of meaning.

Popular psychology is in the process of obscuring the way to a realistic appreciation of illness by a 'cult' of meaning. It must surely be related to a dominant feature of the present culture wherein scientific excellence is able to explain life's phenomena with conviction, but is forcing on our attention a corresponding absence of meaning. Effective definitions and convincing explanations of causes create a false sense of security in the belief that illness – not *an* illness, but eventually illness itself – can be conquered, even if the ultimate moment of death remains, perhaps temporarily, an unavoidable certainty.

This attitude has in many circles undergone a change since the arrival of a depth psychology with a religious dimension included in its constitution. It has curtailed some of the intellectual arrogance with the reminder that 'illness is an essential part of human existence, shadowy and undesirable but nevertheless here to stay.' The novelty – for such it has proved itself to be in psychological circles – that illness far from being a meaningless blemish is in fact a singularly meaningful feature of life, is all that was needed to catch the fancy and swing attention to the other extreme. Illness now has meaning and has joined the ranks of fairy tales, horoscopes, the I Ching and Tibet.

But where does the notion of illness being meaningful come from? Presumably the ancients who saw it as a gift of the gods – or at least as both caused and cured by the same god – cannot have been averse to this notion, even if vague as to its importance; taken for granted rather than reflected. Freud was more directly responsible than religious bodies, Christian or otherwise, for drawing attention to meaning in illness through his insistence on the symbolic factor in conversation hysteria. It intimated a new importance for the role of symptoms that, indirectly furthered by the psychology of C. G. Jung, has become a preoccupation of psychologists.

Jung's influence derived from the more precise recognition he gave to the symbol in clear distinction from the sign, and especially from drawing attention to the meaning it contains as the expression of primordial patterns; the symbol as language of the archetype conveying meaning. The effect of this feature central to his psychology has been enormous, backed by the observation that about a third of his cases did not suffer from any definable neurosis, but from the senselessness and aimlessness of their lives. In his writings on psychotherapy Jung implies that the aetiology of neurosis rests largely on the absence of meaning in life.

His observation that 'a psychoneurosis must be understood ultimately as the suffering of a soul which has not discovered its meaning' is particularly poignant in catching the imagination of many readers and followers. Symbols have caught on. No longer conversion hysteria alone, but all other symptoms and signs of disease have shared the fate of fairy tales and dreams in being recognised as symbols and raped of meaning. The approach, in spite of good intent, has passed a crossroads with a wrong turning that leads back to the point of departure. The hunt for meaning, like the hunt for chemical antidotes, ignores the significance of illness and those who are not intent on eliminating illness now submerge in its symbolism. Both attitudes are highly suspect.

Illness bears a resemblance to the dream in that it is a representation of myth and an experience of immediate significance for the patient. To dissect it for the recognition of universal symbols may bring some intellectual satisfaction, even educational gains, but, in that demand for meaning, the significance of its being is lost. Reason for the oversight is not hard to find, although carefully avoided. For the unmistakable, unacceptable reality of illness is that of a meaningless onslaught, a disaster of major or minor proportions inflicted apparently on an unsuspecting and undeserving victim. Any deliberate hunt for meaning in this experience must detract from its existential importance as a meaningless, undesirable tragedy, with all the pathos and tribulation that tragedy carries. In other words the meaning of illness – if it may be stated in terms of seeming contradiction – is not to search for meaning and turn disaster into good effect, but to withstand and to grapple with the meaninglessness of the tragedy. Better it were to recognise illness in the light of truth as the 'base metal' it is than to gild it with borrowed robes lest in terms of drama the tragedy go unrecognised and appreciation be reduced to the level of comedy. In effect illness is not seen in this light and its tragedy is deemed intolerable. Meaninglessness is suppressed and to that end meaning is sought and applied. But this manner of denial has serious repercussions in the province of healing.

Whether on the side of patient or physician, if we are involved in illness, we are involved in tragedy as surely as those in the plagues of the Old Testament or the chorus of ancient Greek drama. Such events do not simply represent the outcome of a human error, but of a divine providence manifesting as tragedy for which mankind neither has nor seeks to have any answer. The blinding of Oedipus, the madness of Pentheus and the afflictions of Job are lost if explained in meaningful terms of human error and guilt. For those victims their state of anguish was the relentless intent of a divine will without consideration for the whims or wishes of mankind. Whatever form the tragedy of illness may take, its significance can only be appreciated when lived like so-called good health after the manner of its dictates. This does not imply a passive capitulation or stoic indifference.

Much as we may like to believe in the inferred promises of chemical research and of health organisations, it is nevertheless the meaningless interventions of illness rather than the abilities of physicians that dictate our state of health. Illness comes and goes; there is no end to it in this life and never will be. After all, when the pangs of illness have passed are we not obliged to live another 'illness' that goes by the name of good health? The experience is less disagreeable, but no less relevant to life's morbidity. Our health fluctuates and a mistake of the healing professions is a failure to realise there is nothing to be done *about* illness even though there is plenty to be done *with* it. For we are, as T. S. Eliot said, '...in a drifting boat with a slow leakage'. Here is tragedy and truth.

Illness is tragic. That disagreeable feature is only too well known though not in itself a quality peculiar to tragedy. The close kinship of real tragedy with illness lies in the divine nature they share that breaks into life like a violent birth, not with the pleasurable surprise of something new, but with the ruthless determination of a force that without hesitation changes an ordered existence into chaos and holds no promise of respite. Whether it be through Hades the raper, Jaweh the jealous autocrat or any other divine epiphany, the collision with human life is the same. Christ, too, mediates tragedy, but here the impact is lessened with the hope of resurrection and redemption not so markedly to the forefront in other religions. The emphasis of Christianity on the gift of divine hope has moved through the centuries away from divinity into a wishful hoping. It no longer recognises the essence of tragedy which now finds acceptance only through the development of mediaeval and later Elizabethan drama. Outside the theatre walls, tragedy is denied its rightful existence, as we can witness in the disrespectful attitude adopted towards illness.

In this connection it is interesting to note that, although tragedy is communicated through drama and often spoken as poetry, it is music which is the art that has always been recognised as bearing its hallmark with a heart-rending power of tone and incomparable resources of harmony and dissonance harping back to the original oneness of nature. Our destiny is to withstand the chaotic onslaughts from this source of contradictory experiences. It can be devastating in the power of its impact. Artificial hopes can never do more than avoid the paradox of the Dionysian delight in the presence of pain common to both music and tragic myth; the tension of dissonance and the near unendurable wonder of the unresolved chord. Novalis was looking beyond the promises held out by the chemical industries when he wrote, 'Every sickness is a musical problem and every cure a musical solution'.

We may ask in the name of therapy and healing what is the significance of illness as a meaningless tragedy? Every established morbidity, whether as cancer, infectious illness or a neurotic disorder, requires attention to its symptoms for an appropriate handling of the patient's incapacity. At the same time every morbidity is an affliction of the soul reflecting the entire being regardless of the deception lying in localised symptoms. In this capacity it sometimes reaches the hands of the psychotherapist or even the specialist known as the analyst of psyche, in which case it is important to bear in mind that the healing as well as the illness arises at the incentive of that entire being.

A danger to treatment lurks if both patient and therapist, preoccupied with symbolism and meaning, fall victim to the seduction of the symptoms and overlook the individual significance of the illness. It is popularly assumed, for instance, that analytical psychotherapy will cure psychosomatic illness like rheumatoid arthritis, ulcerative colitis or even cancer. It does not. The expectations for cure of symptoms are high and the results abysmal, if not actually dangerous. It does sometimes happen, however, that movements of healing occur during analytic therapy in the course of which it sometimes happens that symptoms disappear; but sometimes not. Focusing on to diseases and their symptoms and crediting them with meaning is no more relevant to the movements of healing than the somewhat similar practice of assigning meaning to dreams and related experiences of the psyche. For dreams – like illnesses – are not to be interpreted and given meaning, but listened to. They share the same mythic background and are the purest communication of tragedy introduced into the body, differing only in the Dionysian violence that thrusts illness on to another level of experience as a physical actuality. In the assignment of meaning, treatment becomes a sort of cure through meaning instead of through medicament.

Tragedy brings home the eternal truth that we cannot dispense with the religious dimension of illness. Yet just that is attempted unwittingly on the one hand by the extremes of scientific expectations and on the other by those of pseudo-religious intents of psychologists. There are occasions when the ruminations of the psychologist's mind are not wanted; when the desire to satisfy, gratify and render meaningful obstructs the workings of the psyche and dictates of the soul. In spite of scientific advancements, illness remains a religious statement referring to matters that cannot be established satisfactorily by physical facts. Most psychologically-minded therapists are at best only dimly aware of this. They overstep their role and fail to see how meaning is something that demonstrates itself and is experienced on its own merit. If this is to be realised in illness it can only be achieved through the acceptance of the inevitable, the inexorable meaninglessness of the tragedy.

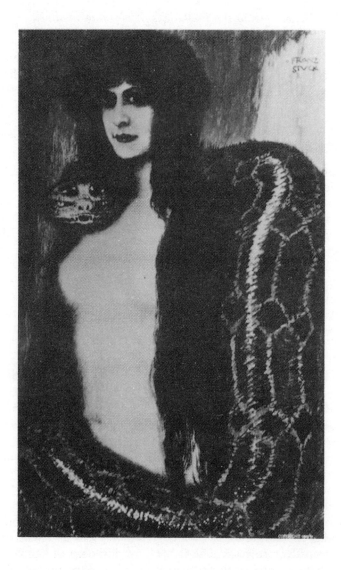

'Sin', 1910, Franz von Stuck, from *Franz von Stuck werkkatalog der Gemälde*, Heinrich Voss, Prestel-Verlag, Münich, 1973

11 · Morbistic rituals

ALFRED J. ZIEGLER

Alfred J. Ziegler is a consultant in psychiatry and psychotherapy. He was trained in psychosomatic medicine, and at the C. G. Jung Institute in Zurich, where he is now a lecturer and training analyst. Influenced by Jung's ideas, he has developed his own 'archetypal medicine', which he sometimes terms 'morbism'. He has run his own practice for many years, in which he has predominantly devoted himself to the psychotherapeutic treatment of physical disturbances. He is the author of *Archetypal Medicine* (Spring Publications 1983) and *Images of a Shadow Medicine* (published in German by Schweizer Spiegel Verlag, Raben Reihe, 1987).

With his poetic exploration of 'archetypal medicine', Alfred Ziegler subverts our assumptions about the 'healing arts' and the 'solar' or 'Apollonian' zeal with which we attempt to annihilate the forces of disease. This chapter, which explores the notions 'morbism' and 'sanism', is drawn from a lecture given at the 1986 Dartington Conference. It should be read with an eye and an ear for image.

Translation by Mark Kidel and Susan Rowe-Leete, with assistance from Reginald Snell.

Attempts to ease the burdens of humanity through medical means almost certainly go back to the dawn of human tradition, and are to be found all over the world. This striving to improve the psychic and bodily well-being of our fellow-creatures is universal: preventively and in response to a crisis, in bloody and gentle ways; by professionals and lay practitioners – orthodox and alternative – through psychological and/or physical means.

155

The self-evident nature of such activity, however, raises the suspicion that this behaviour might perhaps not be entirely conscious, intentional and voluntary. We perceive the helping professions as engaged in an endeavour to promote greater well-being, but this is perhaps only part of the story. We may advance the hypothesis that this universal therapeutic drive involves an archetypal passion, a religious ardour more powerful even than ourselves – a primitive instinct which compels us to treat, even when it might not be entirely necessary. From dietary choices to heart transplants, we are clearly under a kind of compulsion, an inner obligation. The therapeutic act is motivated not just by external necessity, but much more through an archetypal force, which comes into play at the slightest hint of an objective reason.

If this therapeutic impulse, however, has unconscious as well as conscious roots, we must speak, not of therapeutic methods, but of genuine rituals. We are dealing here with 'sacred acts'. In fact, if we follow the history of therapy as well as therapeutic case-histories, we get the impression that this collective passion for therapeutic activity has, more or less autistically, expressed itself in ever-changing forms. It is as if these universal efforts were not just aimed at an objective goal – the amelioration of human well-being – but were directed much more towards appeasing this passion. In our attempt to explore this complex passion, and give it the kind of structure that might be appropriate to a cult, we might propose the diagram opposite.

From earliest times, therapeutic activity has been guided by two principles: on the one hand by the principle of *contraria contraris*, i.e. therapeutic means which counteract or oppose the patient's condition or character; on the other hand of *similia similibus*, i.e. therapeutic methods chosen for their compatibility with the patient's condition or character. These two principles appear respectively in the upper and lower halves of the diagram. And as both allopathic and homoeopathic modes of therapy can equally use psychological and physical means, the model has a right and left side. Most forms of therapy can

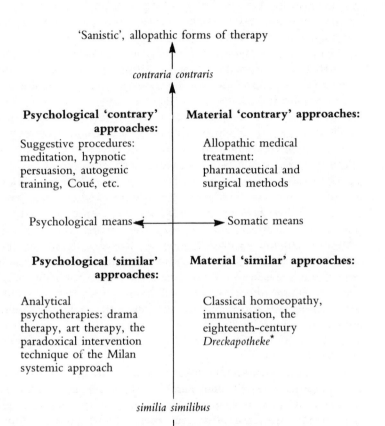

'Sanistic', allopathic forms of therapy

contraria contraris

Psychological 'contrary' approaches:

Suggestive procedures: meditation, hypnotic persuasion, autogenic training, Coué, etc.

Material 'contrary' approaches:

Allopathic medical treatment: pharmaceutical and surgical methods

Psychological means ← → Somatic means

Psychological 'similar' approaches:

Analytical psychotherapies: drama therapy, art therapy, the paradoxical intervention technique of the Milan systemic approach

Material 'similar' approaches:

Classical homoeopathy, immunisation, the eighteenth-century *Dreckapotheke**

similia similibus

'Morbistic', homoeopathic forms of therapy

---

* *Dreckapotheke*: lit. 'dirt pharmacy', a phrase used by the eighteenth-century German physician Paullini to describe the folk and medical use of human and animal excrement in treatment.

therefore be classified in something like the following way:

1 *Psychological 'contrary' methods*: including all more or less suggestive measures, such as shamanistic magic, hypnotic persuasion, certain forms of meditation, Coué exercises, the prayers of Christian Science, autogenic training, and many other practices.
2 *Physical 'contrary' methods*: including the strictly allopathic procedures of medical practice; surgery and pharmaceutical practices whose aim is likewise to treat the disease by opposing it.
3 *Psychological 'similar' methods*: to this belong above all many psychoanalytic practices, therapies based on self-expression, active immunisation and desensitisation and perhaps the so-called *Dreckapotheke* of the eighteenth century.
4 *Physical 'similar' methods*: including classical homoeopathy, active immunisation and desensitisation and perhaps the so-called *Dreckapotheke* of the eighteenth century.

Although therapists tend to have a particular inclination, it is hardly ever the case that they devote themselves exclusively to one of these methods. A psychoanalyst might, for instance, pat his patient on the shoulder and send him, when it seemed appropriate to a surgeon or specialist, or even give him a homoeopathic remedy.

According to this view, allopathy and homoeopathy represent two mutually – but neutrally – opposed forms of medical practice. It is as if we could choose one or the other at will. But in fact we choose between these predilections in a most fundamental way. Each is served by a different sort of person and involves, to some extent, the worship of two quite different god-images; each contains and reflects a fundamentally different creed. The allopathic and homoeopathic therapeutic approaches are therefore more fully described respectively as 'sanistic' and 'morbistic'. These terms express the existential and archetypal differences between these two therapeutic inclinations.

We should not be disturbed by the introduction of yet more unfamiliar terms. They are used here in order to stress the idea that medical methods are also religious cults. This terminology performs a certain task, in much the same way that Latin does in Catholic ritual. The terms 'sanistic' and 'morbistic' have the task (as Latin does in the church) of drawing us towards those religious dimensions which are no longer those of the secular world.

I am not sure if the word 'sanistic' is a neologism or whether it appears in the medical world. I suspect not. 'Morbistic' certainly does not appear in any dictionary. However, it seems to me that the very sound of these words facilitates a perception of the quasi-religious differences outlined above: 'sanistic' has a wide range of associations with all that is healthy; 'morbistic' with all that is 'morbid'. Illness and the diseased can conjure up an image that is on the one hand alien and on the other fascinating.

But let me define this more closely: 'sanism' and 'sanistic' are connected with the Latin *sanare* – to make healthy, to heal, to bring to one's senses. From this derives *sanitas* – health, and *sanus* – healthy. We normally take it as self-evident that our image of health should be 'sanistic'. In any case, nearly all manifestations of the contemporary pursuit of health, whether professional or lay, are embedded in this sanistic definition of health. The sanistic image of health is sacrosanct, an idol which is served worldwide at great expense through preventative and therapeutic endeavours, and re-inforced at all stages of training.

This image of health – which displays its power so self-evidently – is defined quite tautologically by the World Health Organisation as bodily, spiritual and social well-being. In purely conceptual terms, this image is difficult to grasp. If, however, we turn to the symbolic world, we recognise this

sanistic image of health as solar. When we want to tell
someone that our health is absolutely perfect, we infuse it with
solar qualities, using such terms as 'splendid' and 'radiant'
(*blendend* and *glänzend*). All the gods assembled in this
image of health originate from a sphere that might be called
'active/creative' and 'solar'. In this image we are confronted
with the later, shining manifestation of Apollo, powerful
Heracles, Helios with his nuclear energies – a whole series of
divine figures from golden Olympus, not to speak of the
deities of the monotheistic heaven!

We hold the sanistic image of health to be self-evident only
because the solar god-images both lead and mislead us. The
WHO issues definitions of health without realising that such
meanings were in fact invented on Olympus and in the
heavens. It is not surprising that our hospitals should be like
sun-temples, and the staff that work there possess all the
qualities of a priesthood of the sun. The ambulance service is
like a heavenly host, and solar miracle-cures are the order of
the day.

This cult has moralistic and highly warlike implications,
with illness appearing as the enemy; disease is to be fought.
For this reason, the later Apollo is also an *Alexikakos*, rooting
out and exterminating all evil. He was also the Apollo of Mice,
because he regarded all that was not solar as vermin which
deserved to be eliminated. His most heroic deed was to
overcome the being who was his complete 'other', the ancient
Python, the snake-like and poisonous monstrosity which lived
in the swamp near Delphi, and threatened the human world.
What applies to Apollo, in fact, applies as well to all the other
sun-gods mentioned.

Just as it appears to us, in the spirit of sanism, that illness is
(not so self-evidently) self-evidently an opponent, so, in the
spirit of morbism, our feelings toward the morbid, perhaps
not so self-evidently (though in fact self-evidently) undergo a
kind of perversion. It is not only that we have an interest in the

'morbid', but rather that we display a liking for it; a fascination emerges.[*]

It is, therefore, this particular fascination which fundamentally distinguishes all morbistic-homoeopathic rituals – all 'similar' methods – from all that is sanistic.

Here again, if we approach the matter in terms of symbols, these prove to be, as we might expect, anything but 'solar'. By contrast, the 'morbid' is afflicted with all the qualities of the earthly/worldly (*irdisch*), even underworldly (*unterirdisch*). It is almost no longer a question of a sacred image, but rather of a simulacrum, an idol whose conception is as diverse in manifestation as it is coherent in underlying form. Its earliest manifestation is in the image of a 'worm', a dragon, an ogre or similar being. It confronts us, therefore, in the form of those reptilian adversaries of the solar that were mentioned above.

How the WHO would recoil in horror! Physically, these beings are malformed and ugly, covered with growths and skin eruptions; anatomically, they are exquisitely malformed, and physiologically, filled with pure poison. As concerns their spiritual disposition, they are considered dysphoric and ill-humoured; pulled hither and thither by hate, rage or panic; or else they lie around gloomy and melancholic, while their spirit muses on the extermination of humanity, and particularly its heroes. Lastly, they do not make for illustrious company: quite the contrary; they dwell, withdrawn and alone, in caves and gorges, where they drift around *inter faeces et urinam*. Yet, they often appear in the history of symbolism wearing crowns and bedecked with gold, silver and precious stones. They do not, therefore, represent morbistic-homoeopathic therapy in an exclusively sinister light.

Strange as it may seem, morbistic-homoeopathic therapy is in many ways similar to a number of other human subversions, whose character reveals itself under closer scrutiny to be no less religious and cult-orientated. The morbistic-homoeopathic

---

[*] 'Fascination' – from *fascinum*, derived from Thracian magic word for 'bewitching'.

spirit is not confined to the medical world: it is also to be found in the realm of theology, with the heretics' dissociation from orthodoxy, and their lust for the 'spirit that denies'.[*] It occurs in philosophy, when sophists and nihilists preach their sinful epistemologies. It appears in aesthetics, with the mannerists' stance against the classical tradition and with their 'pathophilic' inclination towards the outlandish, the bizarre and the monstrous. Last but not least, it is also to be found in a widely ramifying tradition in ethics, originating with the cynics' rejection of conventional morality. All these are connected, at root, with a fascination for this idol of godlessness whose inspiration is as horrible as it is marvellous.

All genuine morbistic-homoeopathic therapy is in this sense radically 'un-solar'. If it is perverse at a merely superficial level we are not dealing with genuine morbistic-homoeopathic therapy – a therapy which enables us to live through the experience of illness fully and wholly, as a legitimate part of the order of things (*Weltordnung*). It is astonishing how illness can appear from the midst of a laboriously upheld 'sanistic' state, in a way that is quite uncanny. Wished for? Hoped for? Yearned after? There are not only miracle cures, but also miraculous collapses into illness.

Without this radical 'un-solar' deepening, morbistic-homoeopathic therapy would be improper. This applies as much to psychological as to physical treatment; to all those methods, or rather rituals, that are referred to here as analytic procedures, empathy-based therapies, psychodramatic practices, and classical homoeopathy. For Hahnemann, the founder of classical homoeopathy, the simile, the poison, the disease, were nothing less than a sacrament and healing agent. All illnesses were, for him, *morbi sacri*, the changing forms of fundamental disorders which he called 'psora', and for which he harboured a furtive inclination.

The morbistic homoeopathic spirit of the so-called *Dreckapotheke* of the eighteenth century must therefore be

[*]From Mephisto's speech in Goethe's *Faust* Part I.

seen as radical and legitimate. The history of medicine does not do justice to these practices. When snake-poison, crushed toads' eyes, scrapings from mummies and, above all, excrement of various origins were used, these were considered to be just as much *materia sacra* as *materia peccans*. The practitioners of the *Dreckapotheke* saw their excremental means as healing treasure, just as the alchemists of the period believed that treasure was to be found in the mud of the streets – *thesaurus in sordide invenitur*. It is, by the way, significant that all these – alchemy, the *Dreckapotheke*, bizarre medical folk beliefs and somewhat later, homoeopathy – were contemporary to the practice of witchcraft. Here too, reptiles, snakes, salamanders, toads and frogs were considered sacred, manifestly in contrast to the solar-sanistic allopathic perspective, and in order to save us from the solar health (*Heil*), which can so easily become an ill-health (*Unheil*).

It is as if these ungodly beings most need to transform themselves into objects of fascination at that very moment when the solar gods' pretensions become total, and in an increasingly all-embracing way, sanism grows into terror. This is the point at which reverence for the solar gods fundamentally changes direction and turns, in existential despair, towards something quite different; when sanism has become completely unconscious of its own meaning, and can no longer see that the health upon which its gaze is so naturally fixed can also entail a condition of genuine existential despair. The more sanistic health is characterised by all the properties of emptiness and nothingness, the more our reverence for health turns into a reverence for the 'morbid'.

Let us now lay theory aside and consider one particular patient. In purely statistical terms this patient's symptoms indicated that her condition might be improved through analytical psychotherapy. She was not only good looking, intelligent and young, but also charming and articulate; she could express with ease what moved her. She suffered, however, from phobic attacks which prevented her from attending seminars at medical school. These attacks were particularly threatening when she had to face an essential examination and her success was at stake. When exposed, she came out in a sweat, blushed, her hands and feet froze, and her knees weakened and began to shake.

Closer observation revealed that these and other similar attacks had increasingly hampered her everyday life and training as a dancer, as an actress, and as a student of psychology. Whenever her talents drew her into the limelight, she could not bear the exposure. Her sense of being at the edge of ruin was now so great that she made a will and entered into psychotherapy.

At this point she dreamt, drew and wrote a great deal and found many ways of expressing her painful situation in words and images. One day she hit upon the idea of concentrating on her shaking knees and yielding to the experience of herself as a person with a disabled knee. She had discovered that it was in fact easier to stand up when she experienced herself as disabled, than when she had to make a continual pretence at being unshakeable. She experienced herself as healthier when she was aware of being ill and incapacitated. She bought herself a pair of crutches, which she soon mastered. Nobody suspected that her affliction might not be genuine. She went to university, and now found it substantially easier to take part in discussions. She enrolled in the preliminary examination course and even applied for an assistant teaching post. In all these endeavours she made a very convincing impression.

Her self-confidence did not come from feeling sure that with such support, she could never fall over, but her self-assurance could now be maintained because she had fully integrated her infirmity. She could not fall further: she had in any case reached rock bottom, with a certain sensual devotion.

Of course, in such circles, she was asked various inquisitive questions about her knee, but she had ingeniously prepared herself for just such an eventuality. After studying relevant medical books she chose a particular knee injury which would normally require specific surgery and a given period of absence for convalescence. She enacted all this with unsuspected expertise.

It should be said that this patient had transformed herself into a genuine 'sham patient', fascinated by her own pathology. She offered herself, as though in self-sacrifice, to a simulacrum, to an affliction as if it were an idol. She identified with all those specifically reptilian afflictions characteristic of animals that creep and crawl. She also lived out a simulation of the epiphany of that monstrous being which represents the opposite of sanistic health.

She came to realise that there could be no question of charismatic exposure in the limelight without a simultaneous consciousness of humility. She realised, in retrospect, that a readiness to fall on her knees guaranteed her ability to stand with strength. She also discovered that she had not chosen a pathology of the knees by mere coincidence: in terms of the history of symbols, it is precisely through the knee that we can best understand humility, as well as the ability to stand with strength. Neither was it mere coincidence that this patient's limping had become almost second nature. She sought its help whenever her self-confidence began to waver. She hung her crutches on the wall of her study as a votive offering and *memento morbi*.

Two things characterise those therapies which tend towards the morbistic-homoeopathic: a personal 'engagement' by the therapist with the condition to be treated, and a 'spiritualisation' of the condition itself.

While, as we have said, the sanistic-allopathic approach strives to keep illness at a distance – to eliminate it at all costs – the morbistic-homoeopathic approach strives for a real engagement, even a fusion with the 'morbid'. The veneration of the simulacrum, the affliction as idol, involves seeking unification in a kind of erotic passion with all that is horrible. 'Pathophilia' engenders a prurient desire for identification with the diseased. It is not easy to understand how human beings can choose a profession which demands so much in the way of human comprehension.

We find something like this in all analytical psychotherapies, where empathy and rapport play an essential role. It is not by any means the case that everyone whose knees threaten to collapse during phobic attacks should be prescribed tranquillisers or relaxation exercises; it is more a case here of a kind of self-infection by the patient, and the treatment calls for a short-circuit or push in the self-same direction. Accordingly, those who train as analytical psychotherapists must complete – or rather suffer – a so-called training analysis. Here the emphasis is placed upon exercising the capacity to 'make oneself as one' with the particular patient. The so-called training analyses exist in order to refine this potential for empathy.

The necessity for personal experience, central to a training analysis, is echoed in classical homoeopathy. Hahnemann understood this as a readiness and ability for self-experimentation. He expected homoeopaths to discover through self-administration the *simillimum*, the poison, which imitates most closely the clinical condition itself, as well as curing it. He was therefore presupposing a self-sacrifice similar to that which the founders of the psychoanalytical schools expected of their students. The readiness for such self-experimentation was remarkable: Hahnemann and his followers attempted, in countless self-poisonings, to discover the properties of each remedy – or rather, poison.

Furthermore, what goes for analytical psychotherapies and classical homoeopathy applies as well to the shamans and shamanistic practices. Firstly, it is commonly believed that those most suited to such a profession are particularly prone to psychic and bodily afflictions. Shamans have always been expected to be in particularly close touch with the 'morbid'. An important part of the shamanistic task consists in searching for the lost soul of the afflicted person. In order to locate it, or in other words, in order to facilitate the necessary empathy with the illness, the medicine-men poison themselves with appropriate substances. In order to bring about the necessary 'short-circuit' mentioned above, they make themselves ill.

Little of this pathophilic inclination is to be found among

those whose therapeutic practice is inspired by a sanistic-allopathic spirit. They do not strive after the mediumistic. They do not undergo self-experimentation, but learn instead through experiments on others or on animals. And they would shudder at the very thought of having to be deliberately infected.

The second way in which morbistic-homoeopathic and sanistic-allopathic therapies differ has to do with the role assigned to spirit or mind. It is not just a matter of pathophilic empathy, but there is also a need for that which is empathetically felt to be 'dissolved'. The morbistic-homoeopathic approach brings into operation symbolisation and de-materialisation – therapeutic qualities which are sought in vain among strict sanistic-allopaths, who prefer the elegant surgical technique, the optimal remedy, the most efficacious formula and the well-aimed eradication. This is done, not with empathy and spirit, but rather with 'fight' and intellect.

This applies as well to the whole range of analytic psychotherapies: to C. G. Jung's analytical psychology, art therapy, psychodramatic activities from Moreno to Perls, and many other practices. In all of them, the 'morbid' takes on a dramatic form, which becomes symbolic: the simulation of a knee injury is not just a striving for a front-line victory over the disease.

Simulation, in the analytic sense, means an identification with the crippled *per se*. Simulation is an example of the simulacrum, of that morbid idol and adversary of all that is divine and solar. In such a way, simulation attains the status of an art – even a religious and philosophical art. As an image, the 'morbid' joins in the round of all those archetypal images which enable us to know the darker aspects of our existence.

We should of course mention here the amplification method devised by Jung. This method 'opens out' and elevates the experience of illness. Amplification is complete when disease joins the good company of mythic forms, and realises its own value. In the amplification of that alarming knee-failure we encounter those religious practices which, through ritual, express dependence and submission to divine will: for the Shakers and Quakers, the shaking of knees is a sign of divine emotion. But the amplification of a knee affliction points also in the direction of politics: the symbolism of the knee is closely connected with social power and authority. A despot forces others to genuflect and his knees are touched when protection is sought. The word 'genuine', from the Latin *genus* (knee) means 'lawful', 'legitimate', 'held on one's lap' (as a father does his child), 'hereditary'.

For Hahnemann and the homoeopaths, it is not just a matter of empathy with an illness, in this case a form of *psora*, but rather of 'tuning' it to another pitch with 'spiritualised' remedies: when he diluted his simillima to such an extent that little more than a single molecule of the original substance remained in the administered liquid, he intended to potentiate rather than dilute. For him this meant a spiritualisation of the remedy, which would become a subtle substance capable of acting metaphysically; it was as though musically attuned to the patient's clinical condition. For Hahnemann, the illness signified a disharmony of the body, and how else might a purely material remedy reach the disharmonious? He saw disease as a 'principle' which had given up its spirit and become 'stupid' in 'corporeality', as he expressed it. The spirit needed to be adequately restored, and the disease-principle had to be imbued with the breath of 'spiritual water' (*Geistwasser*).

In this, Hahnemann and the homoeopaths were undoubtedly in tune with the romantic philosopher Schelling, for whom a medicine had to be spiritualised (*geistartig*) in order to be effective.

In short, everything that tends towards morbistic-homoeo-pathic therapy, by means of attempts at identification and spiritualisation, becomes absorbed into the service of fasci-nation, in the service of that idol, that simulacrum whose mythological representations are wholly sick, heretical, sinful, and, in terms of the history of symbols, frequently of a more or less reptilian and alien character. It is reflected in our spirit:

we make it the subject of poems, songs, paintings and performances. Its cult knows countless forms of ritual.

We might wonder why these morbistic-homoeopathic inclinations do not irrevocably darken the nature of those that yield and follow them. Why are these people not from the outset dragged down into melancholy, mental derangement and illness? A peculiar incest calls for its own particular eroticism, the same eroticism which seduced the sophists and nihilists in philosophy, the cynics in ethics, the mannerists in art, those whose behaviour in society is considered scandalous, the heretics and Satanists in Christian doctrine, and so on. As the understanding – and hence scope – of sanistic-allopathic treatment becomes more superficial, the fascination for this eroticism deepens. There develops a form of therapeutic nihilism, which does not despair at the incurability of diseases, but rather at the monotony engendered by a particular treatment principle. The eroticism of morbistic-homoeopathic inclinations promises a dark metaphysical pleasure.

Thus a dark erotic experience enters into the incest of morbistic-homoeopathic rituals; the encounter with the primeval principle of illness (*das Urkranke*) involves, to a certain extent, a sensual pleasure. This brings us to the Tree of Knowledge and to the biblical story of the Fall and the intertwining of the serpent and Eve. Above all, this mythological complex entails a break with the solar order and thus also with the dominant sanistic-allopathic principle, which can degenerate so much into boredom. At this point however, we inevitably grasp Aesculapius' snake-staff in our hands; the staff around which a snake winds itself. It is obvious that this caduceus represents the mystical unity of the sanistic-allopathic and the morbistic-homoeopathic, the more so because this same snake is always associated with Hygeia, whom we might well regard as an Eve of Greek mythology.

Thus morbistic-homoeopathic therapy always includes a

further, gnostic element; an element which made heretics of the Cathars in the Middle Ages. It seems that they revered the Grail as the holiest of holies; the Grail or chalice that held the blood of the Saviour. It was made of stone from the crown of Lucifer. The Cathars were nearly exterminated under the Inquisition during the Albigensian Wars, but this did not more to eliminate the morbistic-homoeopathic spirit from the world than did Apollo's or Hercules' deeds. It is not, therefore, surprising that a later descendant of those heretics, the deformed painter Toulouse-Lautrec, should have received this spirit in a new heretical, even sinful way. Toulouse-Lautrec did not tire of painting the whores in the brothels of Paris: those establishments which lie at the margins of the city, in which the 'morbid', deadly infection and sensual pleasure were combined.

And so, the smile of the elderly Hahnemann, in contrast to the seriousness-of-old-age displayed by his sanistic-allopathic colleagues, became as proverbial as that of the aged and chiaroscuro Rembrandt. It is said to be a smile of arrogance, of wisdom and of folly. And it is not unlike the smile of the ancient Roman soothsayers who examined entrails. It is just as hermetic and, I believe, it encompasses the full irony of the morbistic-homoeopathic spirit. It is of autumnal serenity; or should one say, of a perverse autumnal serenity?